Healing the Heart from the Inside Out

Roy F. Small D.O

HERE TO A HEALTHP
BODY, MIND + SPIRIT
Roy

TABLE OF CONTENTS

PREFACE

I dedicate *Healing the Heart from the Inside Out* to my great grandchildren whom I may someday hold but may never personally reach. Through the ages, understanding passes from generation to generation through education, culture, family, and wonderful traditions; however, each individual seems cursed to understand the mysteries of life on their own. It's my hope and prayer to lay a foundation which doesn't have to be recreated in each successive generation; and by building on it, one may move into greater creativity and experience true joy and peace!

"They shall not labor in vain, or bear children for calamity; for they are the offspring of those blessed by the Lord, and their descendants with them" Isaiah 65:23.

"For I will pour water on the thirsty land, and streams on the dry ground. I will pour out my spirit on your offspring and my blessing on your descendants" Isaiah 44:3

INTRODUCTION

Healing the Heart from the Inside Out comes from my heart and I pray it touches yours! The word 'heart' has multiple definitions: ranging from our physical beating heart, to the metaphorical center of all we are; thus, the often-quoted phrase, "I love you with all my heart." Truly, heart is our center physically, mentally, and spiritually. Anthony Hoekema (1994, p211) tells us heart is even the "center and source of all man's religious, philosophical and **moral** activities." As you will see, the word heart also epitomizes holistic medicine. We cannot heal our lives until we heal our heart.

Physical heart disease remains the biggest killer in our country. However, the ultimate source of many forms of heart disease, like most physical ailments, stems from mental and spiritual heart disease. As a Family Physician, walking along side patients for over 25 years, I've discovered four topics concern us most: understanding mental health, overcoming pain, disease prevention, and graceful aging. As you read though these chapters, applying concepts found in medicine, psychology, and theology, you'll learn holistic principles for success in these, and other areas of life.

The first two chapters present a revolutionary view of human nature. Without this understanding, *Healing the Heart* becomes just another self-help book. Drawing from the disciplines of neurophysiology, psychology, and the theological study known as The Doctrine of Man (body, mind, and spirit), I develop a new paradigm for human nature. Empowered with this new concept of self, we're positioned to achieve success!

Although chapter 3 considers the topic of depression, our goal is defining and achieving true mental health. Likewise, chapter 4 investigates opioid abuse and addiction; but ultimately, presents a complete understanding of the nature of pain & suffering, and how to overcome it. Chapter 5 applies this new human nature paradigm, providing practical advice on continually upgrading diet, exercise, and lifestyle. Finally, in chapter 6 we look at aging, which can become a nightmarish situation. However, there are ways to manage and slow the aging process, shortening the gap between health span and lifespan. This information is invaluable as mankind ages and society prepares for its greatest battle.

Each chapter can be read individually. However, the chapters build upon themselves as we move from understanding mental health, to overcoming pain, onto disease prevention, and culminating in graceful aging. Each chapter ends with the subsection, *Moving from Principle to Praxis*: "Praxis is a Greek word that means 'action with reflection'" (Vella, 2002). Praxis is action based on the strength of our built-in principles! *Healing the Heart from the Inside Out* was developed to bring about total lifestyle transformation. To help in this important transition, I employ the concepts of *Transformative Learning*. "Transformational learning is about change – dramatic, fundamental change in the way we see ourselves and the world in which we live. Unlike informational learning, which refers to 'extending already established cognitive capacities into new terrain'" (Merriam et.al., 2007, p.130). The adult education principles of transformative learning fill the gaps in our struggling health care system by assisting people to make the fundamental changes needed for a healthier lifestyle and onto graceful aging.

An underlying theme unfolds in each of the four major topics. I discovered many people become trapped in mental illnesses and/or trapped in chronic pain. I expose how we can even stumble into physical metabolic traps which promote weight gain and inactivity. We'll also explore an epigenetic trap, as we consider aging. Another underlying theme developed as the book came together. Each chapter reviews literature on brain health: how to preserve and promote cognitive function, which allows us to step out of these multiple traps. The age-old question, "are we a product of nature or nurture," resolves as we develop "nous" (the Greek word for 'mind'). We step out of the nature and nurture traps, only as we develop and protect nous. Developing and protecting our mind and spirit allows us to step out of genetic and environmental bondage.

Finally, I've added three appendices. A holistic healing and wellness process cannot ignore spirituality. I take spiritually out of the hand of mystics & theologians; placing it properly, into the hands of common people in the first appendix: "For the Atheist and Agnostic." As noted above, I've developed a revolutionary view of human nature. This new paradigm may seem confusing, and for some theologians, may even seem like heresy. Therefore, appendix two, "For the Theologian and Cognitive Scientist", provides proofs for these new concepts. Not only does 2nd appendix present a new view of human nature, but also, describes a new model for understanding the mind-brain interaction. To balance out the big words and high ideas found in the first two appendices, I've included appendix three, "For the Child at Heart." This 3rd appendix is an allegory to help apply information found in the book.

CHAPTER 1

THE DISCOVERY OF MIND AND SPIRIT

"You have pierced our hearts with the arrow of your love, and our minds were shot with the arrows of your words" St Augustine

A tremendous amount of money and research effort is spent trying to learn what motivates people to prevent disease. Attempting to come to some conclusions, American Heart Association researchers reviewed over 70 individual studies on disease prevention and published a Scientific Statement in the journal *Circulation* (Artinian, Nancy et al., 2010). Among their conclusions, "cognitive-behavior strategies are an essential component of behavior change intervention. These strategies focus on changing how an individual thinks about themselves, their behaviors, and surrounding circumstances and how to modify their lifestyle."

Let's take a moment and consider their findings. What do they mean by **cognitive strategies**? Cognition means thinking. They're suggesting you can improve your overall health and wellbeing by learning to *structure* your thinking: controlling your health by controlling your thoughts. The traps I referred to above (the traps of mental illness, pain, and harmful lifestyles) are only released when we step out of them by controlling our thoughts and structuring our thinking correctly. We're about to set the stage for a way of thinking, an intellectual *environment*, which best controls pain and is most conducive to mental health; a way of thinking which promotes disease prevention, allowing us to age gracefully – all by learning to structure and control our thinking. Beliefs truly do set the thermostat our behaviors revert to.

Next, the researchers suggest **changing how an individual thinks about themselves**. These Heart Association researchers, looking at 70 studies on disease prevention, discovered the importance of understanding who you are. As you come to understand who you are your thinking changes, your actions change, and you're able to overcome health struggles, all by understanding who you are! This is ***Improved Health by Understanding Self.***

Let's look at words used to describe 'self'- who we are – human nature. As I studied psychology I became interested in words like mind, thoughts, emotions, and imagination. I went into medicine and studied the brain, the cerebral cortex (for thinking), and the limbic system (for emotions). Naturally, as I entered seminary training, I became interested in words like soul, spirit, and the metaphorical heart.

I discovered many of these words are referring to the same thing. They all had different names, but, are often referring to the same process. Psychologists talk about psychoanalysis (psycho is your thinking and they're analyzing it – thinking about your thinking). Other psychologists prefer cognitive therapy. The word cognitive, again, means thinking; they're encouraging you to think about your thinking. Medical science deals more with the brain and the prefrontal cortex, the part of your brain concerned with executive function (higher level thinking, decision making and organization). As my training progressed into health education I discovered adult educators talk about metacognition. "Meta" means beyond and cognition is thinking; therefore, metacognition is "beyond thinking", setting back and reflecting on your thoughts.

Ancient writers didn't understand the prefrontal cortex (many thought the brain was just the bone marrow of the skull); rather, they used words like soul, spirit, and the metaphorical heart. Interestingly, for many ancient writers, spirit often meant a higher level of thinking. They may not have understood the brain but that didn't mean they were ignorant. There's still something we can learn from ancient writers about human nature. However, too often people hear the word 'spirit' and get turned off, assuming I'm referring to some religious concept.

Spirituality must not be neglected. Viktor Frankl said, "The spiritual dimension cannot be ignored, for it is what makes us human." Understanding the importance of spirituality, healthcare researchers have tried to give us a less opinionated definition. This is the National Consensus-Derived Definition of Spirituality: "Spirituality is an essential element of humanity. It encompasses individuals' search for meaning and purpose; it includes connectedness to others, self, nature, and the significant or sacred" (Puchalski, et al., 2009). This definition is very broad embracing religious and secular beliefs, as well as philosophical and individual cultural practices, which are so varied in our "melting pot" society.

"Neurologically, we may be designed to search for meaning," says Dr. Miriam Grossman in her book *Unprotected* (2006), referring to research using PET scans which defined "neuronal spirituality circuits." The word 'spirit' can even be used in a very scientific way. What would you name the structure you "sit on" and look back upon yourself and analyze your existence? The word spirit is the proper name for that cognitive 'structure': this is how self-awareness occurs; understanding self-awareness is very important, because increasing it increases self-control and self-motivation.

Every year our nation spends billions of dollars treating and preventing heart disease from the **outside in**. Medications are taken from the outside to change the inside. Catheters probe and scalpels cut through the outside to get inside. Pills can be expensive, catheters dangerous, and scalpels painful; yet, this seems to be all modern man understands. However, our physical heart can be reached painlessly and safely by treating mental, emotional, and spiritual *heart* disease! Indeed, many physical conditions can be prevented and treated by having a healthy *heart*. Words like "heart, spirit, soul, and mind" are often tossed around interchangeably, and yet, they do have very specific meanings.

Before we explore these abstract terms, let me share a story with you. Helen Keller, at the age of 19 months, was struck both blind and deaf. She tells us her teacher, Ann Sullivan, brought **humanity to her life** by teaching her words spelled out on her forehead or hand. The first word Helen learned was "doll." Words for physical objects were easy for Helen to understand but the word 'love' was very difficult to get across to her, until she learned there were words for ideas or cognitive processes. One day Helen was struggling to string beads in a pattern (1 large and two small beads) and getting very frustrated. Ann stopped her and wrote on her forehead the word 'think' (Keller, 1980, p.30). This opened a new world for young Helen, as she understood some words are not about physical things but about the unseen. From there she could move on and understand the meaning of the word love. I'm about to define some abstract words, which lead to abstract concepts, but these are very important because our **beliefs bubble out into behavior**.

The Heart Association researchers suggested we must understand who we are, before helpful behavior change occurs. To better understand terms like mind, spirit, and heart, let's take a journey from the physical to the metaphorical heart. It's easy to see how the physical heart functions. We know the heart is a muscle and it's clear how it performs the function of a pump. The kidneys cannot be understood until you examine them on a microscopic level and see the millions of little nephrons which filter blood. The function of brain and mind cannot be understood simply looking at it or even visualizing the billions of nerve cells with a microscope.

The brain and mind can only be understood by viewing it from yet **another level**, a "spiritual level" (This *emergent* phenomenon is developed further on pages 31, 35 and appendix 2). Once again, I'm using spiritual in a nonreligious, in fact, scientific way. The structure you're "sitting on" when you look back and analyze your existence is spirit. I'm simply adding a new psychological term;

filling a void in the current psychological nomenclature. For those theologians who place added value to spirit, please do not become frustrated, I'm not degrading spirituality but simply lifting the value of our thinking to the spiritual realms where it should be (see Appendix 2: *For the Theologian*).

Healing the Heart from the Inside Out

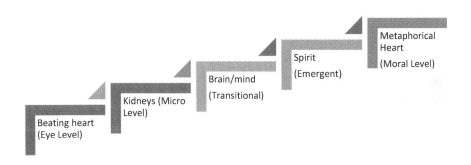

We've almost completed our journey into the center of self; going from the physical heart to the metaphorical heart. Starting from the visible pumping heart we moved into the microscopic and then onto spiritual levels, and now, we're at the metaphorical *heart*. *Heart* adds moral emphasis to our spirit (thoughts, emotions, and will). *Heart* supplies morality to our thinking and emotions, but also, determines the ethical conduct of our will. Just as our physical heart gives life to our bodies, our moral *heart* gives life to our spirits. Spirit creates awareness but *heart* (morality) increases it!

The concept of spirit is empty, it signifies that you're thinking, but it doesn't tell you about the content or the morality of those higher thoughts. Your ethics and morality (the quality of your thinking) is extremely important to your health. Morals and ethics create conflict which makes us grow. In our pursuit to increase self-control, by self-understanding, it turns out this definition of heart is the most important, because adding morality to thinking, opens our eyes. Morality increases self- awareness, morality increases mental strength which, in turn, increases self-control, to overcome bad habits and develop good healthy ones!

Whether we appreciate it or not, we all add some degree of morality to our spirit, which actually increases consciousness. *Heart* is our **conscience** and increasing our conscience increases our **consciousness** (see Appendix 2: *For the Cognitive Scientist*). Adding morality creates conflict and out of conflict arises increased self-awareness. This principle is well known in psychological literature. Sigmund Freud suggested adding morality (superego) to selfish drives (Id) will create conscious self-awareness (ego). Georg Hegel echoed how this occurs philosophically in the concept of dialectic. He used the term **thesis,** the initial state of affairs (here referring to mind/spirit). **Antithesis** (*heart*), challenges thesis and the tension between the two resolves into **synthesis** (consciousness), a new situation (Magee, 2001, p.159). Saint Augustine suggests there can be no separation of purification of the heart from illumination of the mind (Sandin, 1987, p.27). Especially intriguing, is how we can take on the **motivating morality** without the guilt of failure because Jesus taught us, and showed us, the concept of **forgiveness**.

The Heart Association researchers came to understand how a healthy metaphorical *heart* is closely linked to a healthy physical heart. We should never handicap ourselves by underestimating our complete nature. Increasing our *heart* (conscience) increases our consciousness. The level of our consciousness and understanding is significant as research proved, "Poorer understanding is associated with higher mortality" (Bostock & Steptoe, 2012). In short, increasing your moral standards increases your understanding, which makes your life longer and healthier!

Before we explore the concepts of body, spirit, and heart further, I want to encourage you to continue this journey into self-understanding. Adult education researcher Lorraine Zinn tells us, "There's evidence from a number of disciplines to suggest a positive relationship between an individual's beliefs, values, or attitudes and the decisions and actions that make up ones daily life." She goes on to suggest, "Psychological theories, though they differ, often draw a correlation between beliefs, values and/or attitudes, and human behavior" (Galbraith, 1990, p40). So, once again, our **beliefs bubble out into behavior**. Before we can change, and develop healthy lifestyles, we must look at our belief systems and analyze our values.

I've suggested spirit creates self-awareness, but, does self-awareness and consciousness occur at the level of the brain or is it something metaphysical, beyond and higher than the brain itself? The answer is probably both. As a child, we're functioning at a brain level, simply responding to inner drives and the world around us, but around the teen years, transcendence occurs and our **thinking can take on a life of its own**. One higher thought merges with another and eventually this thought world gives **birth** to 'spirit', which allows us to look back upon ourselves and have self-awareness and consciousness. The more transcendent your thinking, the less you're a product of simple brain chemistry, reacting to the world in and around you.

Those who study child development call this higher level of thinking 'formal operations,' which starts to develop in our teen years, when we're capable of thinking about things we cannot see. When we deduce and reason, something 'spiritual' happens, our thoughts take on a life of their own (see Appendix 2: *For the Cognitive Scientist*). Something new develops when your thinking reaches a higher level which doesn't occur dwelling just on the things of the world or yourself. Initially, our spirits lack structure, but life is purposed for developing spirit, developing a spiritual world, a world of ideas. **More importantly, spirit is the 'structure'**

which gives self-awareness and consciousness.

Over the ages people have struggled to understand man's complex physical, mental, and spiritual nature. Words like **trichotomy** are used to divide man into three parts: body, soul, and spirit. **Dichotomy** divides man into a material body and nonmaterial soul. Problems arise as people always seem to place value on one part over another. Too much spiritual attention leads us to neglect our bodies, resulting in physical illness and premature death. Likewise, focusing only on the material world, neglects spirit and reduces power for living. So far, we've considered our spiritual lives, but much of this book deals with the importance of our physical health. However, we'll never be physically healthy until we're mentally and spiritually healthy. A correct "Doctrine of Man" values our physical nature as much as our spiritual lives!

As we study this philosophical and theological material we cannot lose sight of our ultimate goal: improved lifestyle which leads to mental and physical health and ultimately onto graceful aging. Medical educator and professor of Adult & Higher Education, Dr. Daniel D. Pratt, writes "Learning is most affected by a learner's self-concept and self-efficacy" (Pratt D., 1998, p49). Beliefs about ourselves, self-concept, do bubble out into behavior. We know what beliefs and behavior are, but what is this "bubbling out" process, the link between the two, and how does this occur?

Spirit is what we fill our mind with. We could consider 'spirit' to be the software of the brain. But unlike computers, **the software of spirit can actually change the hardware of brain** (this is part of the "bubbling out" process which changes brain, body and then health). This begs the larger question: "What software, spiritual material, is best for creating a healthy mind, brain, and life"? Putting aside all doctrinal and religious views, the historical Jesus and his introduction of the Kingdom of God, is the best "download" which "bubbles out" into complete health and healing. Kingdom of God thinking creates the best intellectual **environment** for growth.

MOVING FROM PRINCIPLE TO PRAXIS

Praxis is action! Moving from principle to praxis is moving with theory into action. What better way to approach total lifestyle transformation then using the adult education principles of *Transformative Learning*, as suggested by its founder Jack Mezirow: "Transformative learners move toward a frame of reference that is more inclusive, discriminating, self-reflective and integrative of experience" (Mezirow, 1997). To make dramatic lifestyle transformations we cannot be afraid of investigating various world views, especially if they're more inclusive of our total life experience and integrates well into all aspects of our lives. "The process involves transforming frames of reference through critical reflection of assumptions, validating contested beliefs through discourse, taking action on one's reflective insight, and critically assessing it" (Ibid, 1997). Mezirow is suggesting we try on new beliefs, evaluate their effectiveness, and apply them into our lives.

In the next chapter, I outline basic Kingdom of God principles; then move chapter by chapter, from principle to praxis (from theory to application). In the chapter *Understanding Mental Health*, you'll see how Kingdom principles create the correct neurological environment to increase frontal lobe function, which prevents, and lift us out of mental illness. As we move into *Understanding and Overcoming Pain*, using the American Medical Associations *Three Hierarchical Levels of Pain*, I show how Kingdom principles take us above ourselves and above the "plane of pain." Kingdom thinking is then applied to *Disease Prevention and Lifestyle*, where you'll see how a healthy brain and mind can correct an unhealthy metabolic syndrome. Finally, in chapter 7, *Graceful Aging*, we discover how Kingdom ideology can even influence your genetic switch setting and slow the aging process. Kingdom of God thinking even, proleptically, infuses aspects of eternal life into us even now!

I defined '*heart*' as morality and, using the theories of Freud and Hegel, showed how morality introduces conflict which increases self-awareness. The Apostle Paul adds another aspect to *heart*; suggesting man cannot 'see' God, or even believe in Him, simply with mind (thinking, feeling or by willing), but it requires 'heart.'[1] I invite those who lack a basic belief in God, or question the validity of the Bible, to read Appendix 1, *"For the Atheist & Agnostic."* Paul tells us our mind, by itself, can never comprehend God! God only shows himself to you through your *heart*. Jesus said, "Blessed are the **pure** in ***heart*** for they will **see** God." God "turns on the light" and relates to us in our *hearts*; thus, the reason for the title of this book *Healing the Heart from the Inside Out.*

Our spirit isn't something nebulous and indefinable, floating somewhere in heaven. Rather, as I've defined it, spirit is inherent within us, even within our thinking. "There is nothing in the bible (nor the main creeds of the church) about disembodied spirits in the next world existing *in vacuo*" (Grider, 2005, p.541). We have a physical body in this life and will have a physical body (though improved) throughout eternity. This places value on our complete nature: physically, mentally, and spiritually. We're human beings and will be human beings even throughout eternity. We're not God or angels, rather just what God wanted us to be, human beings with both a physical and spiritual nature.

Christ, in the form of Jesus, honored our physical nature by becoming one of us, and honored our spiritual nature by giving us His Spirit, the Holy Spirit. Therefore, throughout this book we'll learn to care for, and honor, our bodies and spirits with utmost respect. Man is created in the image of God. This image is best seen in our ability to think and reason. God is very interested in your thinking! Not only are we Homo sapiens, 'thinking beings', we are also children of God! We are the off-spring, the children, of the Most High and Holy God. Think for just a moment what kind of behavior

---

[1] 2 Corinthians 4:6, "For God, who said, 'let light shine out of darkness,' made his light shine in our ***hearts*** to give us the light of the knowledge of God's glory displayed in the face of Christ."

that belief bubbles into.

When the bible uses the word spirit it's often referring to the structure (the intellectual environment), which enables humans to perceive (thought & emotion) spiritual matters and respond (will) to spiritual stimuli (Erickson, 1998, p539). The teachings of Jesus promote the development of higher thinking and spirit, to such a level, it actually takes on a new life. The change was so dramatic, Jesus called it being **born again**. The biblical phase "born again," refers to the birth of a new spirit, **a new life in your mind**. Once born again, spirit takes on new character and dignity; the person, previously incompetent in spiritual matters, is now *made* 'spirit' (Packer, 2005, p1000). By saying the person is *made* "spirit" suggests the overwhelming effect this "new birth" has on an individual. You'll learn how this new, born again spirit, will give you power to overcome negative influences and habits and form new supportive ones!

Being born again occurs after a decision is made. Understanding the infinite perfection of God, we look back upon our own imperfection, and suddenly realize our inability to stand before His consuming glory without help. Once this imperfection is acknowledged, we can make the decision to ask Jesus into our "heart." Finally, we acknowledge Jesus as the Son of God (a term Jesus held to be equivalent with God). He took our imperfections onto Himself and nailed them/Him to a cross.

Before we move on let's look at one last term, 'wisdom.' **Knowledge** is facts and information. **Intelligence** is the ability to acquire facts and information. **Understanding** is the ability to manipulate those facts, to twist them around, and come up with conclusions. **Wisdom,** however, is what we do with those conclusions. Wisdom is how we *apply* all the facts and information we understand.

We all learn a lot of facts and are drenched with information in school, but life itself is constantly presenting us with information.

What is your understanding about life itself? The fact you're alive is obvious, but have you ever twisted this information around and come to any conclusions about it? More importantly what wise applications have you applied to your conclusions about life?

You could skip the next chapter and go right into disease prevention, how to lose weight, how to avoid and treat pain and depression, and how to age gracefully. But I'm afraid, if you skip the next chapter, this book would turn into just another self-help book or just another diet. The next chapter is about the best kind of thinking, the best spirit, which will heal your brain and life! It would be very **wise** to carefully read and understand the next chapter and "download the software"!

CHAPTER 2

KINGDOM OF GOD DOWNLOAD

Men sigh for the wings of a dove that they may fly away and be at Rest. But flying away will not help us. "The Kingdom of God *is within you.*" Henry Drummond

Life was changing: people were losing not only their jobs, but also, their homes and many there lives. Jerome said, "The whole world perished in one city." Rome existed as the center of civilization for over 1000 years. However, in 476 AD, Rome was defeated by the Goths. Many fled to North Africa where a man named St Augustine was ready for them.

Augustine wrote his book, *City of God,* in response to life changing devastation occurring all around him. Using Kingdom of God principles, Augustine was able to reach out to these people in need, as he categorized them as part of the City of Earth (Civitas Terrena) and those of the City of God (Civitas Peregrina).[2] The wonder of Augustine, however, was his personnel journey to be **"otherworldly in the world"** (Brown, 2000, p.324).

Augustine was a master of metaphor and analogy. He looked back to sojourners removed from the original City of God on earth. A city which existed in a garden, toward the east, in a place called Eden. It was there a family made the original decisions. One son decided to build the first city, the city of 'man on earth'. Another son longed for the City of God, which he found in his longing, in his hope, in his thinking. Augustine said, "My **heart** is restless until it finds its rest in thee." Indeed, our spirit, our thinking, must have a

---

[2] From the Latin word peregrinatus: "to travel abroad, be alien," figuratively "to wander, roam, travel about" (Online Etymology Dictionary)

proper dwelling place, a proper intellectual environment, to define and structure it. Jesus gave us the **Kingdom of God, to structure our spirits**: thoughts, emotions, and will**.** The Kingdom of God is not just "the kingdom to come" but also "where Thy will is done." Jesus, proleptically, brought aspects of the ultimate Kingdom to earth.

Augustine challenged the displaced Roman citizens to be less concerned about the human city they were losing, and rather, long for the City of God. **It's this path, from the city of 'man on earth' to the 'City of God' which concerns us now: the path of wisdom!** Jesus introduced an intellectual environment, a spirit, to help us on our journey to the "Kingdom of God."

The foundation and largest collection of Jesus' teachings, we find quoted by His disciple Matthew (an eye witness), and laid out for us at the beginning of the New Testament. Truths concerning the Kingdom of God are recorded in this lecture; truths which will change your life! In fact, the first sentence of this essential teaching is, "Blessed are the poor in spirit, for theirs is the Kingdom of heaven." Here, in one sentence, Jesus puts together the entire doctrine of man I developed in the last chapter, which should now make perfectly good sense. The Kingdom of God is a perfect fit for a poor, weak, unstructured spirit. The Kingdom of God provides the perfect structure to a thinking world! Interestingly, Jesus begins and ends his first lesson with information about the Kingdom of God, a structure used for emphasis, Matthew 5:3-10.

Jesus' teaching concerning the Kingdom of God can be trusted as the word of God. After His baptism and wilderness training, the first words of Jesus recorded for us are, "The time is **fulfilled**, and the kingdom of God is at hand" Mark 1:14. It's very clear Jesus fulfilled the prophecy found in the bible book of Daniel chapter nine. However, Jesus fulfilled not only the *special revelation* found in scripture but also fulfilled the *general revelation* found in history and philosophy. In 500 BC there were biblical prophets such as

Daniel but in 400 BC there were also philosophical "prophets" such as Plato. It's said "Aquinas obtained the 'scientific' **equipment** for his own intellectual synthesis from Aristotle, but received the **substance** of his 'wisdom' from Augustine" (Sandin, 1987, p.28). Jesus fulfilled the biblical and philosophical prophecies of a thinking world.

The Kingdom of God, or what Augustine called the City of God, could be thought of as a '**spirit program**' you may choose to download into your mind; thus, the reason we need to be assured, as noted above, the program is the product of a loving God. Human beings are preloaded with basic 'software', to know God in a general way and to comprehend moral values, but Kingdom of God software is extensive. One could think of our inherent spirit, we have from birth, as something like the original DOS program and the Kingdom of God similar to 'Windows'; it controls and improves upon the DOS program.

The download could be likened to a computer virus but *unlike* a virus, the Kingdom of God download, is helpful mentally and physically. However, *like* a computer virus, it does change *your* program as it slowly eats away at 'self', that part of you that wants to hold onto a decayed and dying world. But remember, Jesus never takes us out of the world. Rather, the download makes us much more efficient, productive, and joyful in the world. Yet, make no mistake, as the song says, "The things of earth will grow strangely dim." Jesus certainly understood the Kingdom of God, on earth, to be in our thinking: proofs for this concept are found in Appendix 2, "*For the Theologian.*"

In the chapters which follow, you'll learn ways to tackle very difficult, seemingly insurmountable, problems such as depression and pain. You'll also learn preventive strategies for cancer and heart disease. However, we can't overcome these obstacles with something as simple as a pill or even a diet. Large life obstacles require an entire lifestyle change. As the Kingdom of God grows you'll develop a sense of wellbeing as it changes your attitude, values, and desires. These Kingdom of God beliefs then bubble out into behavior.

The Kingdom of God download begins as a **decision**. You must allow God to perform this work in you. It begins when you are "born again." We use the phrase "born again," as the spiritual download soon becomes so extensive **a new life** begins to grow. Jesus explains the initial download as a mustard seed which, when a man plants in the garden of his mind, grows into a tree. However, like yeast a woman mixes into a large amount of flour, it soon infiltrates and becomes a part of us; it influences our entire life, not just spiritually but mentally, physically and socially as well.

Why did Jesus use the concept of a Kingdom? It's not so much an analogy as it is a reality. The reality of life is that of God's Kingdom. Many countries like the idea of a democracy, where we all get to vote about rules and laws. However, eternal laws and universal truths are different; they're not part of a democratic system but part of a Kingdom with a King, and you & I are not it! Life is not God's democracy! God is sovereign; He's the King of a Kingdom we call the universe! Years ago, a kingdom was defined, not so much by its borders; rather, by the extent of the king's authority. A king ruled only as far as his authority reigned, only as far as his kingdom had influence. Likewise, the Kingdom of God only extends as far as God has influence in the *hearts* of men.

Indeed, the Kingdom of God is not just an analogy. Other kingdoms have tried to set themselves up as authorities, and in doing so, committed treason. We only need to open a newspaper to see the effects of the kingdom of darkness. Satan has developed a very real and powerful kingdom (a kingdom of lies, accusations, temptations, and ignorance). Satan also enticed man to develop the 'kingdom of self' (a kingdom of pride, greed, and absorbing rather than reflecting Gods glory). Man was never created to live apart from a relationship with God. Satan also joined with us to form many of our social and political structures, the 'kingdoms of man on earth' or what Augustine called the City of Earth (Civitas Terrena). Earthly kingdom's ultimately result in fear, worry and a sense of slavery. We are called to '**die**' to self, '**overcome**' the world and remember Jesus '**defeated**' Satan. Jesus is our King, not just because He's God, but also, because He earned the right. We must determine each day where our allegiance lies.

Jesus never set Himself up to be a political revolutionary and neither should we! "A Spiritual kingdom doesn't need support by physical force" (Guthrie, 2005, p.1061). Remember, our spirit is **freed from any physical connections;** including reliance on social and political structures, common to the kingdoms of this world. However, spiritual kingdoms are involved in spiritual battles and kingdoms can collide. Jesus said, in Luke 16:16, we must forcibly enter the Kingdom of God. The Kingdom of God must be intentionally, purposely, passionately, pursued, and entered into, anew each day. We must establish our rightful "Thinking Place" in the spiritual Kingdom (see appendix 3 "*For the Child at Heart*"). Various commentators have used terms like, "single minded commitment" when referring to our entry into the Kingdom. We need to "seize it" with "fervency and zeal." We must "strive to enter…we must run and wrestle and fight" to have it "upon any terms."

The sun comes up anew each day, and we should daily renew our allegiance and commitment to the Kingdom of God. Each new day truly is the beginning of eternity, in this way time turns into eternity. We enter the Kingdom of God anew each day until finally, one blessed day, we shall enter it anew once and for all.

Behavior change, Jesus teaches throughout His first lecture, must begin in your thinking; it's in your attitude, in your *heart*.[3]

---

[3] Matthew 5:21-22, "You have heard that the ancients were told, 'You shall not commit murder'…."But I say to you that everyone who is **angry** with his brother shall be guilty before the court." Likewise, referring to adultery Jesus says in verse 28, "everyone who **looks** on a woman to lust for her has committed adultery with her already in his **heart**." Thinking was just as important to Jesus as actions. In fact, Jesus implies before these comments, in verse 20, this higher area of thinking is the "Kingdom of Heaven"!

Once again, Jesus leads us away from physical constructs, including behavior, into a spiritual kingdom of motive. You'll never be successful in changing behavior until you're successful in changing the way you think and feel about that behavior.[4] Beliefs bubble out into behavior. The Kingdom of God download changes our *heart* and puts in us the desire and hunger for change.[5] Any behavior change which doesn't begin in the **heart** is destined for failure. Remember, *heart* adds the moral dimensions to spirit, increasing our strength for change! We must develop a "hunger" for healthy living before we can be successful at it. "Blessed are those who hunger and thirst for righteousness, for they will be filled" Matthew 5:6.

It's interesting how this makes perfectly good sense to some people, so valuable to their lives. To others, it's too "unreal, deep, and impractical," or "not what's happening with me today." Jesus told us we **cannot even see** the Kingdom of God until we are "born again" (John 3:3). For those who take time to understand and apply Kingdom of God concepts, they find it immediately applicable to their entire lives. Those who set their mind only on the things around them and ignore spiritual matters are more susceptible to disease and death, but, those who concern themselves also with spiritual matters are healthier and more alive. In order to live peacefully and successfully we must keep our minds on spiritual things and live in the Kingdom of God!

We may be able to <u>see</u> the kingdom, but Jesus tells us in Matthew 18:3, unless we humble ourselves and become like children we will never <u>enter</u> it. Not only must we have faith but we must have **childlike faith**. Not only must we trust but we must have **childlike trust**. Learning to let go and trust God is hard because it makes us vulnerable, but remember, God is strongest when we are

---

[4] 2Cr 7:10, "For the sorrow that is according to the will of God produces a repentance without regret, leading to salvation, but the sorrow of the world produces death."
[5] "Sonship leads to likeness and inheritance." Cameron, W.J., *Evangelical Dictionary of Theology*, ed Walter Elwell, p440

weak!

We've developed a concept of being "grown-up." We train up our children as if something magical happens at age 18 or 21. The truth is, we never arrive at some grown-up state, rather, life should be viewed as a "journey." How joyful when we quit trying to be grown-up and learn to humble ourselves as children. How joyful when we learn to run to our Heavenly Father, as we did to our earthly parents, when scared and things in life were in total disarray.

King Jesus is not teaching submission but rather trust. The alternative is to struggle through life on our own, with no help from God, which turns out to be the most dangerous situation of all! The most challenging patients I've encountered are the elderly, who've struggled through life on their own. After years of struggling alone, they become very cynical and angry, as they never developed trust in God. Jesus tells us not to worry about food, drink, or shelter - like the people who live in the 'kingdoms of this world'. Again, spiritual kingdoms don't depend on physical resources. We cannot ignore life on earth but we should "seek first His kingdom and His righteousness, and all these things will be given to you as well" (Matthew 6:33). It's a matter of priorities. This verse tells us to seek first His Kingdom but also **His righteousness**. Jesus refers to "His" righteousness not ours! He didn't come to condemn us but to save us.

MOVING FROM PRINCIPLE TO PRAXIS

Transformative learning theory suggests the process of 'perspective transformation' has three dimensions: psychological (changes in understanding of the **self**), convictional (revision of **belief systems**), and behavioral (changes in **lifestyle**) (Transformative Learning, 2017). In chapter 1 we discussed the importance of understanding **self**. Here, in chapter 2, we saw the importance of **belief systems**. Finally, prepared with these psychological and convictional tools, it's time to take the first behavioral step in your journey into a dramatic **lifestyle** transformation!

Jesus' most important teaching on the Kingdom is found in John 3. Please do not **harden your heart** but carefully follow His path of wisdom from "your kingdom" to the Kingdom of God.

> Jesus replied, "Very truly I tell you, no one can **see** the kingdom of God without being born again." "How can anyone be born when they are old?" Nicodemus asked. "Surely they cannot **enter** a second time into their mother's womb and be born!" Jesus answered, "Very truly I tell you, no one can **enter** the kingdom of God without being born of water and the Spirit. Flesh gives birth to flesh, but the Spirit gives birth to spirit."

Jesus says you cannot see, let alone enter, the Kingdom without being **born again**. You were born once into this fleshly kingdom but you must also be born again into a spiritual kingdom. None of this will make sense until you make a decision to be "born again" and invite the Kingdom of God to be downloaded into your mind and become your spirit!

I would invite you, even today, to say an age old prayer which has turned around the lives of countless people over the centuries. In this prayer you admit, like all mankind, you've gone astray from Gods plan and, like all mankind, need to be reconciled (brought back) into the presence, care, and protection, of this most High and Holy (set apart) God. You must acknowledge Jesus died on the cross for you, to pay the price you are unable to pay for treason committed to His Kingdom; the price for trying to set up your own kingdom in defiance of God's Kingdom. You must acknowledge Jesus is the path of wisdom and the only way back to God.

If you believe, please pray with me, "Jesus, I believe you're God's only begotten Son and you took the punishment I deserve for treason committed to Your Kingdom. I now ask for forgiveness and ask that I may be a part of your Kingdom. In Jesus name, amen." The bible says, if you believe with your ***heart*** and confess with your mouth Jesus is the Son of God you will be saved! You've believed with your *heart* but you must also confess with your mouth: confess with your life journey. No one can walk the path of wisdom from the kingdom of self to the Kingdom of God alone. You must get in contact with a trusted friend or spiritual leader and tell them you made this decision and need the help of a community of believers!

CHAPTER 3

UNDERSTANDING MENTAL HEALTH

She had endured much at the hands of many physicians, and
had spent all that she had and was not helped at all, but rather had
grown worse. Mark 5:26

The remainder of this book will review four major life obstacles
and reveal practical applications of the holistic principles we've
developed. Remember, we must understand mental health before
the next chapter on overcoming pain. Likewise, disease prevention
is next to impossible if struggling with pain and pills. Finally,
successful aging requires all three areas function well.
Understanding mental health requires an understanding of our
complete nature as human beings: physically, mentally, and
spiritually. The physical world is easier to understand, being
investigated with our 5 senses; however, our mental and spiritual
environments are sometimes difficult to comprehend, often resulting
in disarray. Therefore, the first two chapters presented the proper
way to organize our mental and spiritual lives to function most
efficiently.

Depression is so common we'll use this condition as a
representative case study; however, our ultimate goal, is to examine
the characteristics of mental health. What does true mental health
look like? Also, understanding depression may allow you to help
someone with the condition. Studies estimate 10% of us suffer from
depression and we have a 10% lifetime risk of developing it. These
statistics are important because inadequately treated depression can
lead to permanent structural changes in the brain. On the other hand,
optimism is a significant predictor of positive physical health
outcomes (Rasmussen et al., 2009).

Improving depression also reduces physical pain. Depression and pain are linked in the brain and can influence one another. Pain can lead to depression; however, depression can lead to, and aggravate, pain. The Annals of the Rheumatic Diseases published a study suggesting depressed mood may be linked to rheumatoid arthritis disease activity. Researchers showed depression was not just a result of pain but high depression scores accurately predicated arthritis flare-up measured 6 months later (Overman et al., 2012).

Depression is also linked to coronary artery disease, one of the biggest killers in our country. Shimbo et al., (2005), showed depression "significantly predicts the risk for first coronary heart disease events." Depression also significantly increases the risk of developing a stroke. In fact, the depression-stroke association is similar to the association between smoking and stroke (Pan et al., 2011). The link between cardiovascular disease and depression is so strong recommendations were made by an American Heart Association subcommittee to elevate depression to the level of an independent risk factor for heart disease; similar to hypertension, elevated cholesterol, and diabetes (Lichtman, et al., 2014).

SYMPTOMS OF DEPRESSION

We're going to begin by reviewing the symptoms, causes, and finally, the treatments for depression. However, let's not forget our ultimate goal of understanding what true mental health looks like. Studying mental *illness* sets the stage for understanding mental *health*.

Depression can have both emotional and physical symptoms. The emotional symptoms are feelings of guilt, sadness, tearful, helpless & hopeless feelings, loss of interest and pleasure, suicidal thoughts, anger & irritability. However, we need to be careful as many of these feelings are a normal part of life. Horwitz and Wakefield, in their book, *The Loss of Sadness: How Psychiatry*

Transformed Normal Sorrow into Depressive Disorder, suggests human sadness and its various forms such as grief, shame, guilt, despair, and anguish are often normal and should not be treated as a pathologic condition. Psychiatrists have tried to clarify what is normal and abnormal in the Diagnostic and Statistical Manual (DSM). However, Dr. Allen Frances, who previously chaired the development of the DSM-4, suggests new drafts "essentially pathologizes normal behavior." Mental health professionals can sometimes take what is normal and suggest it maybe a disease.

Increasingly, people are going to be labeled depressed or diagnosed with some other "pathologic disease." Ultimately, we need to understand what real mental health looks like! After all, much of what we call mental health is just "constructed" cultural standards, and many people are labeled ill, when they're just different, or have difficulty fitting into societies ridged routines and expectations of what they think is normal. Mental health also keeps us physically and spiritually healthy; but, what does true mental health look like? Too much attention is placed on what's abnormal and not enough on what is normal.

Depression often presents with physical symptoms: lack of energy, decreased sex drive, changes in sleep and weight, excessive concern over physical health and even pain. Depression is also associated with cognitive problems: anxiety, obsessive rumination, brooding and worry, decreased concentration and memory and even pseudo-dementia. Everyone experiences memory problems as we age; but, pseudo-dementia presents with profound concentration and memory problems, even a cognitive decline, and turns out to be due to a treatable condition like depression. Sometimes getting the right medication to the right person can change their life! This is important to understand, especially as I go on to discuss alternative or additional treatments for mental illness. I'm not against medications; don't stop a prescription without consulting your healthcare provider.

It's sometimes helpful to break depression into two subtypes:

outside (exogenous) depression and an **inside (endogenous) depression**. People with "outside" depression have life stressors a pill may not help and may even worsen. However, people with "inside" depression often respond well to medications. I want to review three simple questions to help distinguish between these two conditions. People with outside "stress induced depression" often have trouble falling asleep (worrying about problems), while those with "chemical imbalance depression" fall asleep ok, there's nothing serious going on, but cannot stay asleep. Stressed out people often wake-up hopeful the day will go well, and then, one problem after another results in a depressed mood. Truly depressed people, however, wake-up depressed and stay depressed all day. Finally, you can sometimes tell the difference between endogenous and exogenous depression by eating habits and weight. Although not always the case, *stressed out* people tend to *stress eat* and gain weight, whereas, clinically depressed people often lose interest in everything (including food) and can lose weight. However, those with outside depression may also benefit from antidepressants, especially if their stressors have been severe and persistent.

Fatigue, often a part of the symptom complex of depression, is sometimes simply a lack of "**passion**." How many times have you been playing a new video game or reading a book and just couldn't put it down? You became passionate about the experience, and along with passion, comes energy. We can sometimes lose passion for life, in general, and develop fatigue. As we explore treatments for depression, you'll discover, spiritual awaking and renewal increases passion for life, resulting in renewed energy. We all need to develop a passion for **life** (see discussion on the numinous found in appendix 1).

CAUSES OF DEPRESSION

Let's look at depression from yet another view – looking at its causes. First, the biological causes of depression, then psychological and social causes, and finally, peering into the spiritual roots of depression. We'll break the **biological** causes of depression into hormonal and brain disorders.

Hormonal changes associated with adolescence, menses, menopause, and the dramatic hormonal changes associated with pregnancy can sometimes lead to depression. Thyroid disorders and low vitamin D can influence mood. Anyone with persistent depression should have thyroid and vitamin D labs drawn. Disorders of the brain, such as a stroke and chemical imbalances, can result in depression. Stroke victims can become depressed due to their loss of function, but also, due to brain chemical changes associated with the stroke itself. Many of these biological causes of depression can be treated with antidepressant medications.

It's not just large strokes that disable people. With the introduction of MRI scans, we're seeing individuals who've experienced numerous tiny strokes, from hardening of the arteries in the brain, resulting in depression and even dementia. Diabetics are particularly susceptible to this vascular depression; and, it's sometimes hard to diagnosis and treat, as the depression is so tied up in their other medical issues. Most importantly, these conditions can be prevented with lifestyle modifications. Obesity, improper diet, and lack of exercise can elevate insulin levels, resulting in high blood pressure, elevated cholesterol, diabetes, and depression: a condition known as Metabolic Syndrome.

Another biological cause of depression is inflammatory chemicals which can accumulate in body tissues. Miller et al., (2009) showed how these inflammatory chemicals can enter the brain and cause depression. Stress, inter-personal conflict, and social isolation can turn on adrenaline and cortisol, but also, the "fight or flight" response of our sympathetic nervous system. Ultimately, this all leads to excessive activation of our immune system and release of these inflammatory chemicals. Simply put, stress leads to inflammation in your body and brain. More importantly, this inflammatory response is going on 24 hours a day in people who are overweight! Even if we're not particularly 'stressed out', obesity results in a constant release of inflammatory chemicals. These chemicals leave the blood, enter the brain, and effect brain cells function, resulting in depression. This is a perfect example of mind-body unity: the condition of our physical state directly affects our mind, and, the things we think about directly affect our body. We cannot isolate the functions of mind and body.

Continuing to investigate biological causes of depression; dysfunction of the brains prefrontal lobes can result in depression (Pascual-Leone et al., 1996). Interestingly, some depressed patients even have a decrease in blood flow to the frontal lobes. The brain is divided into four lobes. The frontal lobe, and more specifically the prefrontal area, is the part of the brain that makes us most human. The prefrontal area is the control center of the brain; involved in behavior planning, decision making, emotional control, and self-awareness (which we've discovered is so important in health), also, the prefrontal area controls morality and spirituality. When the prefrontal area is not functioning correctly we experience impairment of moral principles, social impairment, lack of foresight, problems with abstract reasoning, loss of empathy and lack of restraint.

Phineas Gage taught us what it's like to live without the left frontal lobe. On Sept 13, 1848 Phineas was working in railroad construction, blasting through rock, when his tamping iron rocketed through his face and out the top of his head. Amazingly, he lived 14 more years. Gages' physician Dr. John Harlow wrote his medical report in 1868,

> The equilibrium or balance between his intellectual faculties and animal propensities seems to have been destroyed. He is fitful, irreverent, indulging at times in the grossest profanity (which was not previously his custom), manifesting but little deference for his fellows, impatient of restraint or advice when it

conflicts with his desires.... In this regard his mind
was radically changed, so decidedly that his friends
and acquaintances said he was "no longer Gage."

The prefrontal lobe of the brain affects our personality, self-restraint, moral standards, and our ability to commitment to family, church, and loved ones.

Dr. Neil Nedley in his book *Depression: the Way Out*, shows how frontal lobe dysfunction and depression are interconnected and influenced by our lifestyle! Nedley points out the frontal lobes give us "**the ability to identify and implement strategies to help alleviate depression.**" Therefore, decreased frontal lobe ability can cause depression; the depression, then, decreases the frontal lobes ability to get out of and alleviate the depression. A vicious cycle develops: as depression worsens so does the frontal lobes abilities to relieve us of depression. **This vicious cycle impairs our natural ability to overcome the depression**. An analogy would be the disease of "Aids." The Aids virus attacks the actual immune cells responsible for fighting the virus. So, depression attacks your **mental immunity**, your immunity against depression, and does so by decreasing your prefrontal lobe abilities.

You can understand how bad lifestyle choices, such as poor diet and lack of exercise, can lead to heart disease, cancer, and stroke; however, these same bad lifestyle choices can lead to decreased brain frontal lobe function. An even larger vicious cycle then develops. The decreased frontal lobe abilities, with loss of behavior planning, loss of proper decision making, loss of self-awareness and self-control, then leads to numerous lifestyle problems, and ultimately, to multiple chronic diseases. These multiple chronic conditions, then, leads to further decreased frontal lobe function.

TRAPPED

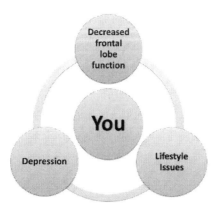

The person is trapped in a vicious triangle: a harmful lifestyle which leads to decreased frontal lobe function and onto depression, which causes the harmful lifestyle to only worsen! People with depression and other mental illnesses are trapped, trapped in a **dungeon,** and many never find their way out! Now that we've reviewed some of the biological causes, let's quickly move through some of the psychological and social problems leading to depression; then, onto treatment, and finally, take a look at mental health.

Numerous **psychological** problems can present with depressive symptoms. People struggling with obsessive compulsive disorder (OCD) are frequently depressed as the condition enslaves and controls so much of their lives. Bipolar disorder, once called manic depression, cycles between depression and mania. In my experience, bipolar disorder is frequently over diagnosed. Those who fail treatment for depression are often misdiagnosed with bipolar. We see this occurring a lot more as drug companies charge an unbelievable amount for some bipolar medications.

Admittedly, bipolar can present in several ways and with numerous variants; so, I'm thankful for psychiatrists to help us sort through these. However, it's hard to miss a true bipolar individual, especially if their manic events are not controlled. Finally, anxiety disorders, panic attacks, and seasonal affective disorder can all have associated depressive symptoms.

Many social problems present with depression because relationships are so important; and, when not running smoothly, can be such a big source of distress. I place substance abuse in this category as it frequently starts, and is perpetuated, in the context of social situations. Introducing foreign substances into the brain can result in endogenous depression (the chemical imbalance type of depression, I referred to earlier) which is difficult to treat using antidepressants alone. Indeed, substance abuse is a big cause of depression and needs to be dealt with before sorting through a lot of other possible causes. Marijuana, in particular, is very 'depressogenic' or depression beginning. Alcoholics are frequently self-medicating depression; and, just as the condition starts as a social disorder, it must be treated as one. People abusing alcohol need to seek and accept help from others, especially Alcoholics Anonymous. Unemployment, both imposed and self-inflicted, can result in depression as people were made to work, and without it, often feel incomplete.

We've looked at the biological, psychological, and social causes; let's turn our attention to the spiritual roots of depression. You'll recall, from chapter one – *The Discovery of Mind and Spirit,* I'm using 'spiritual' in a nonreligious, in fact, scientific way. Spirit, a world of thought, **emerges** as one thought merges with another. Eventually, this thought world takes on a life of its own, giving birth to 'spirit', allowing us to look back upon ourselves and have self-awareness. The ability to develop spirit occurs during the "formal operations" stage of cognitive development; usually in our teen years. Spirit is the 'structure' you're sitting on when you look back and analyze your existence. Spirit is the cognitive 'structure' which gives self-awareness and consciousness. Author Paul Davies (1983) writes about this **emergent** phenomenon,

> In the case of living systems, nobody would deny that an organism is a collection of atoms. The mistake is to suppose that it is nothing but a collection of atoms. Such a claim is as ridiculous as asserting that a Beethoven symphony is nothing but a collection of notes or that a Dickens novel is nothing but a collection of words. The property of life, the theme of a tune, or the plot of a novel are what have been called '**emergent**' qualities. They only emerge at the collective level of structure, and are simply meaningless at the component level.

In summary, your thoughts "emerge" from your brain and cannot be **reduced** simply to brain chemicals. Brain cells and brain chemicals, like musical notes or words, come together collectively, like a symphony or novel, and thoughts "emerge" - that's spirituality!

John Ratey, in his book *A Users Guide to the Brain* (2001, p140), brings together various theories of how consciousness develops, writes "Somewhere in between these two positions is the idea that the mind is an emergent property of the brain – it is what results when the brain runs." Reductionist thinking (reducing thoughts to brain chemsitry) is fine when attempting to understand physical systems; but, higher human thinking takes on higher spiritual meaning.

Some readers may be thinking, "There he goes again, writing about all this mind, brain, psychobabble, 1960's stuff." How does this apply? Just as there are biological, psychological, and social causes of depression, there are also spiritual roots of depression. Along with the stage of formal operations, comes certain 'cognitive needs', which are not met dwelling on just the things of the world or yourself. Failing to acknowledge and attend to spiritual development contributes to a sense of aimlessness, resulting in feeling overwhelmed, helpless, and hopeless!

Thoughts centered only on the things of this world or ourselves, often end up as depressive thoughts. Sarah Young, in her book *Jesus Calling*, seems to agree with this. Referring to "renewing your mind", she writes "When your thoughts flow freely, they tend to move toward problems" (Young, 2004). Embracing spirituality allows us to take every thought, emotion, and motivation captive. Spiritual development is the scaffolding, we climb on, to look back and reflect upon our lives. Spirituality allows us to understand, control and change our thoughts, mood, and motivation. Spirituality enables and inspires us to change!

To summarize the causes of depression. First, we looked at biological conditions: hormonal, metabolic, and brain problems. We then investigated psychological causes including anxiety, OCD and bipolar. Social problems such as relationships, employment issues and substance abuse can lead to depression. Finally, we turned to the spiritual roots of depression, such as, dwelling on ourselves and the world around us, and not taking every thought captive.

TREATMENTS FOR DEPRESSION

Now we're going to review biological and psychological therapies, then onto spiritual treatments for mental illness. We'll be concentrating on depression, because it's so common; however, the principles apply to other mental disorders as well. Don't forget, our ultimate goal is to understand mental health!

"She had endured much at the hands of many physicians, and had spent all that she had and was not helped at all, but rather had grown worse" (Mark 5:26). While this bible verse is not referring directly to mental illness, it could be, as multitudes have received various treatments for mental illness and have only grown worse.

Mental illness is a devastating problem, and can be difficult to treat; therefore, it must be understood and managed holistically: body, mind, and spirit.

Before we evaluate specific treatments for mental illness, we must look at overall **lifestyle.** Is your lifestyle conducive to healing, is it fertile ground? It's almost impossible to treat depression without adequate **exercise.** Researchers from Duke University showed a moderate exercise program reduced depression as well as antidepressants (Blumenthal, 2007). **Proper diet** is essential to your wellbeing. Numerous studies have shown a lower incidence of depression and anxiety in vegetarians compared to nonvegetarians. You need adequate **rest**, relaxation, and sleep. Appropriate **social interactions** are invaluable. Many people with mental illness tend to isolate themselves, which only makes things worse. We all need a sense of belonging and family. I can't emphasis enough the importance of just **getting outside**: it's hard to "see" God inside man-made structures. Are you drinking enough **water** or is your brain shrunken from chronic dehydration?

What are your **stress reduction** techniques, do you have any **spiritual disciplines**? What are you filling your life with? What are you **filling your brain** with? Are you watching horror movies or sad, depressing programs? What about obsessing on news programs? Of course, we need to avoid **drugs and toxins**; even caffeine, but especially alcohol and tobacco. Smoking one pack or more a day results in a threefold increased risk of major depression. It's hard to treat mental illness, with specific therapies, if our overall lifestyle is not conducive to healing. How effective is dropping a Prozac seed into the garden of your mind, if it's full of weeds and thorns?

First, we'll look at some biological treatments for mental illness. Transcranial Magnetic Stimulation, thought to increase prefrontal lobe brain activity and blood flow, is used for certain types of depression. Electroconvulsive or "shock therapy" can be very effective in treating resistant depression, even in the elderly, and done humanely under general anesthesia. Light therapy and vitamin D are often used for Seasonal Affective Disorder. Herbal supplements are sometimes helpful. Of course, there's a pharmacopeia of prescription medications for mental illness, all having 'biological' effects.

If thoughts are an **'emergent'** or spiritual phenomena, why are physical treatments, like antidepressants, effective? I've developed an analogy, called ***Light Bulb of the Mind***, to understand the effect of medications. Mind could be thought of as a light bulb. A light bulb transduces electrical to light energy. The mind transduces the electrical energy of the brain into the "light" energy of thought. Brain, mind, and thought are three distinct entities. The brain, with trillions of electrochemical interconnections, could be thought of as the electrical supply to the bulb. Mind should be thought of as the actual light bulb (transducer) and thoughts are the "light" emitted. **Thoughts are as different from brain as light is from electrical activity.** 'Mind' is altogether different from brain and thoughts. Mind is an "organ", created by the brain, from which thoughts 'emerge' (see appendix 2, *For the Cognitive Scientist*).

Medications for mental illness could be thought of as a **dimmer switch,** increasing or decreasing electrical supply to the bulb, or a **toggle switch** changing the color of the light. Medications can change the brightness or color of thoughts but will not control them! Medications will never take a negative, sad, destructive thought and turn it into a positive, happy, productive thought – only you (your spirit) can do that. Again, the amazing thing about the whole process; the 'light' of thought can take on (give birth to) a **whole new life**, so complex we give it the name "**spirit**"!

Our brain cells and brain chemistry only give us the capacity for emotions, thought and will (motivation); therefore, medications only alter that ability, but do not control, our actual feelings, thoughts, or desires. How do we get control of feelings, thoughts, and desires? For that we'll need to look at psychotherapy's and counseling.

The field of psychiatry, with their medications, is attempting to "reduce" mind and thoughts to brain cell circuitry and brain cellular chemistry. Medical science made amazing advances **reducing** disease to the microscopic level. Understanding biochemistry and molecular biology, allowed researchers to develop miracle drugs to treat all kinds of conditions; such as, infections, cancer, arthritis, and heart disease. Therefore, society pushed psychiatry to follow this same 'reductionist' model to treat mental illness. Society pushed psychiatrists to "find a pill for it." Thoughts, however, cannot be reduced to the biochemical level. Neuroscientist, Niall McLaren (2010) explains it this way,

> **Reductionism** (reducing thoughts to brain chemicals) has failed to give a human account of mental disorder, leaving a huge intellectual and *moral gap* that holistic medicine is best suited to fill...science questions empirical (observational) facts, but it does not question logical truths. It is a logical truth that the experiences of tasting beer, struggling with a math problem, and feeling grief are not properties of molecules but are properties of a highly ordered system.

To put all this in perspective; medications, dietary supplements, electroconvulsive and light therapies could be considered **reductionist** therapies. People who rely solely on these treatments believe depressive thoughts and feelings are the result of an abnormal brain – they reduce thoughts to the brain level – and try to fix the brain. However, other therapies are considered "metacognitive." Meta means beyond and cognitive means thinking. Therefore, thinking about your thinking, is metacognitive; the basis for psychotherapy's, cognitive therapy, self-help, education, and spiritual therapy's.

Not all depression is biological, therefore, psychologists are experienced in a variety of counseling methods. Cognitive Behavioral Therapy (CBT) is very effective for depression and proven to be just as effective as medications for panic disorder. CBT is thinking about your thinking. Patients learn to identify emotions and "automatic thoughts", including engrained unproductive ways we deal with life, they also learn to identify and analyze common misconceptions. Cognitive therapy helps us step back from ourselves and look at specific emotions, thoughts, and behaviors. Therefore, I consider cognitive therapy to be spiritual therapy. I know these abstract ideas maybe tiresome, and sometimes hard to understand; but, that's the reason there are so many depressed people!

Beck and Rush (1988) suggests mental illness is a result of systematically biased information processing. CBT identifies and corrects thinking (cognitive) distortions and specific, habitual errors in thinking. They suggest "the way in which individuals **structure** their experiences determines how they feel and behave." Merriam et al., (2007, p346) tell us the ancient Greeks were fond of thinking **categories** and used them as the basis for discovery. Christianity provides thinking structures or categories for true self-discovery, allowing us to play good with others, and function well in the world around us.

Too often our thinking lacks structure**,** therefore, we can't control it. Patients often tell me, "I can't turn my brain off at night; one thought leads to another." Our thinking (spiritual) world, lacking physical structure, cannot be seen; so, people tend to ignore it, and that's where the problem lies. To simplify things, and learn to structure our thinking, psychologists have developed the idea of schemas.

Schemas are broad mental categories, almost like storage bends, we put things in. Schemas develop automatically over our lives and help us make sense of everything. Referring to these "knowledge structures," Merriam et al., (2007, p 401), suggest "Schemas are not just passive storehouses of experience, however; they are also active processes whose primary function is to facilitate the use of knowledge." Hopefully, our thought structures are helpful, and not harmful, to ourselves and others!

Beck and Rush suggests schemas are enduring cognitive structures; **thinking themes**, which develop and can "influence subsequent concept formations" (they grow and develop). Schemas are also involved in reality testing. Therefore, if your life theme is abnormal, you can lose the ability to view things objectively, and even start believing lies (which is the scariest 'place' of all). It's not just people with mental disorders, who've learned abnormal ways of processing or structuring thoughts and information, we all do to some extent. A depressed person, or maybe someone who's just struggling with a bad mood, at some point, must get control of their thinking!

Cognitive therapy, helping us think about our thinking, leads us to a plane higher than ourselves; therefore, could be considered a form of spiritual therapy. Just as we can hire professional organizers, to put our possessions into storage containers; over the century's, people have tried to develop preprogramed ways to structure thinking. Worldviews are prepackaged schemata. Worldviews give us preset patterns to organize our thoughts, so we can live life, and not constantly worry about analyzing it (suffering the, so called, paralysis of analysis).

Reductionists suggest a pill can change our brain chemistry, which changes our thinking, to achieve mental health. Conversely, the **metacognitive** view, suggests the things you think about can change your physical brain, and along with that, your life and health. A simple electroencephalogram (EEG) shows how things you think about, your state of mind, can change the electrical activity of the brain. This is like software changing the hardware; it doesn't happen in computers, but it does in your brain. Neuropsychiatrist John Ratey (2001, p17), suggests the brain is malleable and transforms itself according to what we learn, think and experience; "experiences, thoughts, actions, and emotions actually change the structure of our brains."

The bigger and most important question: what kind of thinking, what kind of schema, what kind of preprogramed worldview, what kind of spiritual program has the best effect on your brain, on your life, and consequently, on your health? Some people consider themselves agnostic; suggesting, they don't have enough information to make a valid overall worldview about "what's going on" and "what it's all about." However, over the century's, some people thought they had enough information; they were the founders of **thinking programs** we call major world religions: men like Buddha, Mohamad, and Jesus.

In the first chapter, I showed the importance of understanding who you are! I showed what "an individual thinks about themselves, their behaviors, and surrounding circumstances" can modify their lifestyle. I've also shown what you think and expect can actually re-shape your brain. **So, what's the best type of thinking**; what's the best thinking program or worldview to improve your life and health?

Jesus designed a spiritual "software" program to get the most out of this thinking machine we call our brain. Jesus lived in a very unique time, blending Greek philosophy & teaching with Jewish religion (see appendix 2 *For the Theologian and Cognitive Scientist*). He presented us a unique way to *structure* thinking for mental and spiritual wellbeing, which ultimately, leads to physical health. The teachings of Jesus persisted through time as they were revolutionary and healing. In fact, the word Jesus used for 'save' is **sozo,** which is translated also into the word "heal or be whole." The salvation Jesus brings includes health: mentally, physically, and spiritually!

How does this apply to mental health? Jesus taught us to value **life itself**, not only our experience of it. Our experience maybe bad, however, life itself is still good. Jesus taught us to think of God as our **Father**, not just some harsh dictator of rules, leading to guilt. He showed us **eternal life** is possible, which brings the ultimate hope. Jesus released us from the bondage of **unforgiveness** (which leads to all kinds of mental disorders). Just as important, Jesus gave a thinking structure called the **Kingdom of God**. He understood thoughts created only by the 'kingdoms' of this *world around us* or those centered on the Kingdom of *self*, often end up depressive thoughts. Our thinking needs the *structure*, only the Kingdom of God can bring. I'm not suggesting brain washing or thought control; simply a proper platform or structure to place your thoughts in; an environment for your personal chosen thoughts to live in.

Ancient writers prioritized thinking into levels: beginning first with the level they called the **flesh**; this includes not only our immediate physical environment but also the events in our day to day life. It's quite easy to build a world around the flesh, as the bricks and mortar are readily available, through our senses. However, the world we live in has become so complex, it overwhelms and overtakes much of our thought processes, leaving what is left in disarray. We can **restrict** our thinking to simple 'cause and effect' by preoccupation with the things and events in this world, or allow our minds to do what it was created for, the development of the magnificent!

Individuals with depression often have **restricted** thinking. A person with exogenous (outside depression), for example, may feel restricted based on finances and responsibilities. A person with endogenous (inside depression) is often restricted from finding pleasure in life, restricted by decreased energy levels, and decreased enthusiasm. Various medical professionals would give their own reasons for this restricted thinking. Psychoanalysts may suggest conflicts in development; whereas, Psychiatrists may suggest improper brain chemistry has restricted the person. The issue, however, is one of cause and effect; did the depression cause the restricted thinking or did restricted thinking cause the depression! I suggest the latter – restricted thinking caused the depression.

What happens when the homo sapien (the thinking being) restricts his thinking to just the world around him? What happens when the homo sapien simply becomes a stimulus response creature, like the animals around him? The ancient writer Jude, who many believe was actually the brother of Jesus, wrote about people who only think about the world around them, what he called "devoid of spirit." Jude wrote, "What they understand naturally, like creatures without reason, in these things they are destroyed."

Henry Drummond, in 1883, wrote about the experience of those so destroyed, who live only in this physical world and fail to develop a spiritual environment. Drummond, in his book *Natural Law in the Spiritual World*, did an interesting comparison of the how the laws of nature control growth and development, in both the physical and spiritual worlds. He wrote about the experience of those who have no thought **structure** (no environment for their spirit to dwell), whose thoughts are only determined by the world around them.

> The moment we pass beyond the mere animal life we begin to come upon an incompleteness. The symptoms at first are slight, and betray themselves only by an unexplained restlessness or a dull sense of want. Then the feverishness increases, becomes more defined, and passes slowly into abiding pain. To some come darker moments when the unrest deepens into mental agony of which all the other woes of earth are mockeries, moments when the forsaken soul can only cry in terror for the living God (p. 118).

We need to stop for a moment because this is painful! Drummond is taking us into the mind of someone who could potentially commit suicide, they've lost complete control; their thinking has no environment or structure.

Drummond writes, "Up to that point the natural Environment supplies man's wants, beyond that it only derides him… Where is the **Environment** to complete this rational soul?" Essentially, he's asking "where is the environment, the structure, for your rational thinking." He goes on, "Men either find one – One – or spend the rest of their days in trying to shut their eyes." Of course, by using the capital "One", Drummond is referring to God. Drummond understood our need for structured thinking. We need spiritual environment as much as we need a physical environment; without it we can feel lost and incomplete! "There, without Environment", Drummond tells us, "the darkness is unutterable. So, maddening now becomes the mystery that men are compelled to construct an Environment for themselves. No Environment here is unthinkable. An altar of some sort men must have – God, or Nature, or Law." So destroyed are those who live only in this physical world and fail to develop a spiritual environment.

As individuals, we're free to construct the content of our thinking anyway we choose. Not even God will interfere with your thinking world, even if the content of your thinking, ultimately, results in killing yourself or someone else. I'm obligated to alert those suffering from mental illness; they may have a potentially life threatening disorder. I've methodically reviewed symptoms and treatments for depression but failed to reveal the extent of suffering associated with it. Depression hurts; however, unlike physical illness, where the end can often be seen, depression seems to have no end, and, for some, may have no end!

KINGDOM OF GOD vs. DUNGEONS OF THE WORLD

Jesus understood the plight of those trapped in the vicious triangle of harmful lifestyles, decreased frontal lobe function and depression. Many people are **trapped** in the kingdoms of this world, in the dungeons of this world, or within themselves. Sadly, many never find their way out! Patients with depression are trapped inside thinking patterns which are **restricted**, closed and unyielding;

trapped inside the dungeons rather than living in the Kingdom. After his baptism and wilderness training, Jesus went home to Nazareth and declared war! In effect saying, "I'm going to set the captives of this thinking dungeon free"! He stood in their synagogue and said, "I have come to proclaim freedom for the captives and release from darkness for the prisoners."[6] To us, these are words of comfort, but to the "Kingdoms of Ignorance and Darkness" they were fighting words, a declaration of war! God was bringing the "Kingdom of Knowledge and Light", the Kingdom of God, to this world!

A morbid preoccupation with self, or the structure and things of this world, results in morbidity (illness). Ancient writers encouraged us to live life on a higher level, to develop a spiritual world. Ancient writers knew the reality of God, and the sense of security and wellbeing He brings to life. Yet, those who "did not think it worthwhile to retain the knowledge of God, he gave them over to a depraved mind" (Romans 1:28).

Breaking out of the dungeons of this world and the shackles of self, is not easy and requires a thinking world with **structure**. Wouldn't you agree the word 'Kingdom' implies structure? Although, ultimately the physical Kingdom to come, Jesus brought aspects of the Kingdom of God to our thinking experience. The complexity of human thinking requires something other than just responding to the world and thinking only of oneself. Jesus understood this and gave us a thinking world, the Kingdom of God. He understood our thoughts need the substantial structure only a Kingdom could bring. As the spiritual Kingdom is constructed, our consciousness is no longer *restricted* to the world or ourselves, enabling us to have victory over depressive worldly thoughts and harmful actions. "For the mind set on the flesh is death, but the mind set on the Spirit is life and peace" (Romans 8:5).

---

[6] Luke 4:18 & Isaiah 61:1. Interestingly the Septuagint interprets "prisoners" as "the blind."

WHAT DOES MENTAL HEALTH LOOK LIKE?

It's safe to say our healthcare system, in general, focuses more on disease than health; this is also the case in the mental health professions. In fact, I don't recall ever seeing a comprehensive statement defining mental health. Using principles we've explored thus far: holistic medicine, doctrine of man and Kingdom theology; we'll develop a view of true mental health.

Before I suggest a formal definition of mental health, I would like to review one of the inspirations behind this book. A medical school professor once commented on a luxury of primary care; suggesting he could refer complicated patients to a specialist. The truth is, people go back to their family doctor when specialists are unable to help. I've found this especially true in the treatment of mental illness. Thus, the practice of medicine becomes an art and not just science; hopefully, an art born out of compassion and not just frustration.

Over the last twenty-five years, numerous patients have walked through my exam rooms in desperate situations; feeling helpless, as no one could find an answer to this depression and anxiety that has so consumed their life. Mental illness is a formidable enemy; man's attempts to conquer the beast often seem fleeting, and quite frankly, just pitiful![7]

Healing the Heart from the Inside Out is not just about healing your physical body through the healing of your heart and soul; but also, opening my heart and life to yours. God only knows how I've struggled over the years to develop just the right words, to go from my heart to touch yours. Although you may not agree with the following definition of mental health, please agree it is heartfelt!

What does mental health look like? Simply put, mental health looks like Jesus. Certainly, this view goes against many cultural standards. Many even thought Jesus was crazy: John 10:20 says,

---

[7] "We have not brought salvation to the earth the people of the world have not been reborn," Isaiah 26:18

"Many of them were saying, "He has a demon and is insane. Why do you listen to Him"". The word "insane" is used four other times in the New Testament, once in Acts 26:24-25: standing before King Agrippa, Paul told his testimony and shared the gospel message. Festus interrupted and said "Paul, you are out of your mind! Your great learning is driving you mad." Undaunted, Paul replied, "I am not out of my mind, most excellent Festus, but I utter words of sober **truth**."

Paul is suggesting truth is the opposite of insanity. Neil Anderson (2000, p.23), in his book *The Bondage Breaker*, says "Freedom from spiritual conflicts and bondage is not a power encounter; it's a truth encounter…Satan's power is in the lie, and when his lie is exposed by the truth, his plans are foiled." Healing comes from simply exposing the lie. Those in bondage, Anderson suggests, are not liberated by a pastor or counselor but "by what they choose to believe, confess, renounce, and forgive." Mental health is living in the Truth (also see page 173).

St Augustine has been called a teachers' teacher; his life permeated by education. "We learn", Augustine suggests, "not through words sounding in the ear but through **truth** teaching us from within. 'By means of words we learn nothing but words.' To get beyond words to their meaning we must depend on a 'knowledge of realities' that we already possess" (Sandin, R.T., 1987, pp 26 & 28). This knowledge of realities or "**disciples of truth**", depend on an internal knowledge which results from "divine illumination." Interestingly, 1 Timothy3:15 reveals, the church is the "pillar and support of the truth."

Healing the Heart from the Inside Out, touts the importance of both a healthy physical and metaphorical heart. I've defined one of the metaphorical functions of the heart to be morality; suggesting morality introduces conflict, which in turn, increases self-awareness (increasing our conscience increases our consciousness). Spirit creates awareness but heart (morality) increases it. Therefore, increasing morality increases our strength for living and improves mental health.

The case could be made, suggesting many depressed people are already burdened under a weight of guilt; so, why increase guilt by focusing on morality? In fact, sometimes well-meaning therapists, friends, and family try to lessen a depressed person's guilt by avoiding moral issues. Neuropsychiatrist John Ratey (2001, p339), reduces guilt by suggesting abnormal brain cells and brain chemistry are the cause of mental illness; this "approach frees them from a great deal of shame and self-blame, as they come to see the neurological origins of their challenges." Could the effect of this rhetoric result in lack of standards; leading the mentally ill person to even use their disease as an excuse for immorality; which, further complicates their life? The truth is, a lack of morality can result in depression. You'll recall Niall McLaren suggested reductionism (reducing thoughts & behavior to brain chemistry) has left "a huge intellectual and *moral gap* that holistic medicine is best suited to fill." The beautiful forgiving nature of Christianity is the answer to this controversy. We can develop moral standards without the accompanying guilt of failure, because, Jesus taught and showed us the concept of forgiveness.

With the principles of truth and morality in mind, we can expand our definition of mental health. You must agree, mental health looks like **correct** thinking or **right** thinking, or better yet, **wise** thinking. There was an old English word for proper thinking: 'right wiseness.' In fact, the word 'rightwise' was used in early English translations of the bible for the word we now use, which is 'righteousness.' The closer we move toward right wiseness; the closer we move toward an understanding of what is right and wrong; the closer we move toward righteousness; the closer we're moving toward true mental health.

As we continue to develop the Kingdom of God as the proper structure for our thinking; Matthew 6:33 tells us to "seek first His kingdom and **His** righteousness, and all these things will be given to you as well." Jesus refers to "His" righteousness not ours! Remember, He didn't come to condemn us but to save us. Furthermore, Romans 14:17 says, "For the kingdom of God is not eating and drinking (cultural things), but **righteousness** and peace and joy in the Holy Spirit" (parenthesis and emphasis added). If we clearly saw and understood our unrighteous thoughts and behavior, we certainly would think it mentally unstable! If, however, you pass Gods test of righteousness (right wiseness) you have true mental health. Real mental health is the righteousness of God, in all times and in all places, it's not cultural. **The righteousness of God is manifest to us in the life of Jesus.**

In summary, I would define mental health as "Retaining the knowledge of the Truth of God, holding universal standards of morality, while living in Righteousness as joint heirs with Christ Jesus." Although I would never be so pretentious, to suggest this statement as the final, comprehensive definition; it is workable, and seems to fit with the apostle Paul who writes, "And just as they did not see fit to have knowledge of God any longer (they continued to suppress the truth); God gave them over to a **depraved mind** (lack of morality), to do those things which are not proper (unrighteousness) " Romans 1:28 (parenthesis & emphasis added).

Understanding mental health as living in the Truth of God and the Righteousness of Christ Jesus, allows us to develop a remedy for mental illness. James wrote, "If any of you lacks wisdom, let him ask of God, who gives to all men generously... but let him ask in faith without doubting" James 1:5-6. Asking God for divine illumination, for wisdom or right wiseness, is important; but understand, what He [God] will reveal to you is Himself. Mental health is understanding who we are as joint heirs with Christ Jesus; heirs of a Kingdom!

MOVING FROM PRINCIPLE TO PRAXIS

Praxis is action! Moving from principle to praxis is moving with reflection into action. It's time to make some dramatic changes in the way we think, see the world, and the universe. Adult education researchers Boyd and Myers (1998) tell us 'discernment' is fundamental to the process of transformation. Discernment is the ability to use rational **insights, judgments, and decisions**; but just as important, are **symbols, images, and feelings** which <u>motivate</u> us. Jesus understood this principle 2000 years ago, when He gave us the insights, symbols, images, and feelings He called the Kingdom of God.

The teachings of Jesus made such a profound impact on people, He called it being "born again." But, once we've been born into this thinking Kingdom it needs "bricks and mortar" to structure it. The "bricks and mortar" of the Kingdom of God are laid down as we develop spiritual disciplines and understanding. Understanding and applying, the "10 Commandments of the Kingdom," developed below, will help correctly structure your thinking to overcome many mental conditions, but also, other life obstacles.

1) The kingdom of God must be entered **anew each day**. It's not a decision that's done once at some alter; but a decision that must be made each day, until one sweet day, we enter it anew once for all eternity. Each day the sun comes up anew: each day is truly the beginning, not just of the rest of your life, but the rest of eternity. In this way "time turns into eternity."

2) The Kingdom of God must be **purposely, sometimes forcefully, entered**. One does not stumble into the Kingdom of God! You must find time at the beginning of each day, no matter how rushed, and declare your intention to enter the Kingdom. Understand, there will be times, the Kingdom must be forcefully entered. Jesus said, "The kingdom of God is being preached, and the people are forcing their way into it" Luke 16:16. There will be times, throughout each day,

when kingdoms collide: the kingdoms of self, the world, Satan, and God. Kingdom collisions are not always obvious, because we're too involved in the experience of it. You can tell when kingdoms collide because you start to feel depressed, angry, envious, or a host of other negative thoughts, emotions, or drives. Indeed, there are times each day, we must stop everything in life and forcefully enter the kingdom! Jesus uses a parable in Matt 13:33, "The kingdom of heaven is like yeast that a woman took and mixed into 50 pounds of flour until it spread through all of it." Most of us can only imagine how difficult it would be to work yeast into 50 pounds of flour; similarly, a difficult job working Kingdom principles throughout our lives (all of it)! We must intentionally, purposely, passionately, pursue the Kingdom of God each day.

3) Each day we need to acknowledge and celebrate **Jesus as our King**. People in democratic societies sometimes don't understand the sovereignty of a king. The king will not be neglected. Your allegiance to Jesus must be declared each day. Are you going to live in, and build, the 'kingdom of self'? Are we going to be slaves to the 'kingdoms of the world', or the 'kingdom of darkness', or declare ourselves, and live as, children in the 'Kingdom of God'? To this you must declare your allegiance each day. God hasn't called us to walk out of the world, but until He does, we do know where our allegiance lies and we know our King walks alongside us.

4) Not only do we to acknowledge King Jesus, but also, **glorify Him**. As we look upon the King we're immediately struck by His glory. It's been said, the first step in confidence is understanding how big God is. If your God's not big, then He's not big enough to care for your life. When we glorify

God, we come to an awareness of his awesome abilities, and develop a renewed confidence in His ability to care for us. The Apostle Paul said, "For although they knew God, they neither glorified him as God nor gave thanks to him, but their **thinking became futile** and their foolish **hearts** were darkened. Although they claimed to be wise, they became fools" Romans 1:21 (emphasis added). Paul goes on and says, "Furthermore, just as they did not think it worthwhile to **retain** the knowledge of God, so God gave them over to a depraved **mind**, so they do what ought not to be done" Romans 1:28. We must acknowledge and glorify our King, but also, **retain** the knowledge and glory of Him throughout the day; it must become a lifestyle!

5) We must **present ourselves** daily and **bow to the King**. Psalms 2:12a says, "Do homage purely to the Son, that He not become angry, and you perish *in* the way". Interestingly, the Greek word for 'way' is 'derek'; which, as I show in the last chapter, refers to **lifestyle**. We are to pay homage purely to Jesus, or we shall perish in our lifestyle. Other translations of Psalms 2:12 reads "Kiss the Son" or "Submit to Gods royal son": this, however, is not just submission, as it lifts us up as well! When we present ourselves to God, we declare ourselves as God's child, a brother of Jesus, and joint heirs with Him; giving us the confidence we need each day. To look upon our King is to be conformed into His image!

6) The King declares **law**. We don't live in the democracy of God. God has declared certain rules and laws we must acknowledge. This is where we lose many people, for two reasons. First, too many believe the kingdom is just about rules and walk out. Second, many stay but live in a state of constant guilt, because they can't seem to follow the

rules. The apostle Paul acknowledged this conflict in his own life and writes: "There is therefore now **no condemnation** for those who are in Christ Jesus. For the law of the **Spirit of life in Christ Jesus** has set you free from the law of sin and death" Romans 8:1-2. An important law to understand in the Kingdom is the law of the "Spirit of life in Christ Jesus." Unlike religious 'kingdoms', the Kingdom of God gives us the right to live as individuals with our own preferences, without guilt and shame; yet, we must acknowledge the Rule of God. Recall, the content of this thinking/spiritual world must have 'heart'! Heart is the values, morals, and judgments we place on our thinking. Conscience develops as values are placed on thinking. A developed conscience then gives us the breath of consciousness to obey the rules. But make no mistake, a spiritual kingdom must have values. Selfish thoughts must be valued less than the wellbeing of others. Anger must be replaced with forgiveness. Obsessive, worried thoughts must be replaced with truth!

7) The King declares **truth**. Truth determines culture: culture does not determine truth. As we look around the Kingdom we are overwhelmed by the light (knowledge) and truth that Jesus gives. The Kingdom of God is the Kingdom of knowledge and truth. The kingdom of darkness is the kingdom of ignorance and lies.

8) We must **trust** our King; knowing he cares for us and will accomplish what concerns us each day. We must not only have trust, but, childlike trust and faith. "Truly I say to you, whoever does not receive the kingdom of God like a child shall not enter it at all" Luke 18:17.

9) Until the Kingdom of God comes in its fullness, there will always be a **struggle** with other kingdoms. We must **die** daily, to the kingdom of 'self'. We must **overcome** daily, the 'kingdoms of this world'. We must **recon** daily, the 'kingdom of darkness'; understanding and acknowledging Jesus' defeat of Satan and his kingdom of darkness. Vine's Expository Dictionary, in referring to the Kingdom (*basileia*) says, "those who enter the Kingdom of God are brought into conflict with all who disown its allegiance, as well as with the desire for ease, and the dislike of suffering and unpopularity, natural to all. On the other hand, subjects of the Kingdom are the objects of the care of God."

10)   The heartbeat of the Kingdom of God is the **heartbeat of eternity**. Kingdom walkers always have an eternal perspective; and, always have tight hold on the "rope of hope" which is secured in the true tabernacle of God, in the true eternal Kingdom!

CONCLUSION

Our spiritual/thinking world requires both structure and content, which regulates both emotion and desire. As the Author of life, Jesus understood this and gave us the Kingdom of God! This view of life fulfills all our mental requirements! Martin Lloyd-Jones said, "The real cure for most of our subjective ill's is ultimately to be so enraptured by the beauty and glory of Christ that we will forget ourselves and will not have time to think about ourselves at all. Now that is a good bit of psychology." Even the "Prince of Preachers", Charles Spurgeon, suffered with depression and ultimately had to put it in the hand of God: "Causeless depression cannot be reasoned with, nor can David's harp charm it away by sweet discoursing's, as well fight with the mist as with this shapeless, indefinable, yet all-beclouding hopelessness. The iron bolt which so mysteriously fastens the door of hope and holds our spirits in gloomy prison needs a heavenly hand to push it back." **May the heartbeat of this King, the heartbeat of eternal life, enter your heart and heal your life!**

CHAPTER 4

UNDERSTANDING AND OVERCOMING PAIN

The torments and suffering in this world are beyond the comprehension of everyone except God Himself. Therefore, anyone speaking of pain, speaks of things they don't completely understand. God spoke to Job and his friends, who were trying to understand pain: "Who is this that obscures my plans (darkens counsel) with words without knowledge" Job 38:2. Nonetheless, this very serious torment to humans must be dealt with, as many live their lives either in constant pain or in constant fear of pain. Suffering seems not only epidemic, but even thought of as part of the human condition. Nothing else in life seems to matter when we're hurting.

Let's explore how pain changes us physically, mentally, and spiritually. Research shows pain can **physically** change your brain. "Chronic pain is associated with reduced brain gray matter and impaired cognitive ability" (Seminowicz, et al., 2011). However, "treating chronic pain can restore normal brain function in humans." Civil War physician, Dr. Weir Mitchell, in 1892 describes how pain changes us **mentally**: "Under such torments, the temper changes, the most amiable grows irritable, the bravest soldier becomes a coward." John Milton in *Paradise Lost* wrote, "But pain is perfect misery, the worst Of evils, and, excessive, overturns All patience." Pain calls our **spiritual** beliefs into question and even reality itself. Indeed, pain distorts reality, and, pain is a reason many deny the reality of God. As a Christian, I have a calling to clear God's good name, as many blame Him for suffering. I'm called to declare the good news: through our belief in God, pain can be controlled. God gives us the directive to "declare that the Lord is upright; He is my rock and there is no unrighteousness in him" Psalms 92:15.

As a physician, my life is often filled with the observation of suffering and the drive to reduce it. However, a very real source of tension has developed in our medical community. Garcia (2013) tells us chronic pain affects more Americans than heart disease, cancer and diabetes combined, and yet, Yokell et al., (2014) suggests prescription opioids are involved in 67.8% of all overdoses. This dissertation on pain is important because pain and pain pills, not only enslave people to the healthcare system, but are also killing people.

The United States is only a small part of the world's population, yet we consume 50% of the world's drugs and 80% of the world's pain medications. Opioids are drugs like codeine, tramadol, Vicodin, Norco, Percocet, OxyContin, and morphine. Our country is eating up 80% of the world's supply of these drugs. Why? No one likes to be in pain – let's take a moment and look at the **experience** of pain through the poetry of Emily Dickenson.

"The Mystery of Pain"
Pain has an element of blank;
*It cannot recollect when it **began**, or if there were a day **when**
it was not*
*It has no **future**, but itself, its infinite realms contain its **past**,*
enlightened to perceive new periods of pain.

As we experience pain, Emily suggests, we're really on a different **plane** of existence; so, it's easy to get lost and even trapped in pain. Thankfully, the tools we've developed in previous chapters can help us stay above the "**plane of pain**" and find our way out. Pain is a formidable enemy but can be overcome by understanding. Pain, especially chronic nonmalignant pain (CNMP), needs to be addressed from a holistic standpoint: body, mind, and spirit. The holistic standard of care was substantiated, by both the Institute of Medicine (2011) and Medical Clinics of North America (2016), as they point to the biopsychosocial approach to treating pain. Before investigating the holistic approach to overcoming pain, we'll look at

'Understanding Pain and the Brain' and then 'Understanding Pain and Correct Thinking'.

UNDERSTANDING PAIN AND **THE BRAIN**

I frequently illustrate the body's natural pain fighting mechanism as thousands of tiny catcher's mitts and baseballs in your brain. Imagine brain cell chemical receptors as tiny catcher's mitts and our natural painkilling endorphins as baseballs. There's typically one catcher's mitt for each baseball and everything is in natural balance. If we experience a painful situation, our natural baseball painkillers fall into the catcher's mitts resulting in pain relief. Now think of opioid pain medications as thousands of baseballs all pounding on one catcher's mitt. As the brain always attempts to keep an equilibrium, it will "down regulate" or reduce the number of catcher's mitts. Thus, opioid pain medications can actually cause pain if not used correctly.

I was nine years old when I had my first real experience with pain. I suffered with an earache for two days, and spent at least one night, agonizing in severe nonstop pain. Toward the evening of the second night grandma cut a Percocet (oxycodone) into a quarter tablet and gave it to me. After a short time, the constant throbbing pain I'd experienced for two days started to die down; and, I was even left with a wonderful sense of **well-being and security**, as I could finally lie down to rest.

Now I can look back upon the experience and understand, from a physiologic standpoint, exactly what happened. Opioid pain killers have two effects on the brain. First, they block the actual pain you feel: opioids block the nerve impulse to the sensory part of the brain. Stimulating the second pain relieving pathway; leading to the emotional and pleasure center of the brain; what I call the "blessed second pathway", can cause **euphoria (a warm sense of security and well-being)** helping us endure the painful condition.

Understanding the two pathways is important, as these same brain centers can be modulated naturally without medications.

In summary, pain has both a sensory component, what you <u>feel</u> as pain; also, emotional, and cognitive components, your experience of pain, which can result in <u>suffering</u>. There's a very real difference between feeling pain and suffering. I believe it was Haruki Murakami who said, "pain is inevitable but suffering is optional." Why do we have this second "blessed" pain relieving pathway? God understands the interaction between pains physical and emotional components! In fact, it's often difficult for us to separate physical and emotion pain as the pathways are closely related in the brain.

Another brain area, used to modulate pain, is the prefrontal cortex, which I referred to in previous chapters. You'll recall the prefrontal brain controls 'executive functions': thought processes that regulate, control, and manage other thought processes, also, regulating **emotions, imagination, and pain**. Emotions, imagination, and pain can all get entangled in the brain. The prefrontal cortex, however, comes to the rescue, allowing us to **untangle suffering**. In reviewing Dr. Howard Schubiner's book, *Unlearn Your Pain: A 28-day Process to Reprogram Your Brain*; John Jerome PhD, explains how "continuous pain and stress reactions can become ingrained in the mind, body and spirit." **The mind, he says, can then twist your body into pain.**

Dr. Gregory Esmer et al. (2010) did research on *Mindfulness-Based Stress Reduction, for Failed Back Surgery*; investigating the thinking of people with chronic pain after back surgery – a very difficult problem to treat. He teaches us to first become aware of pains physical component, and then, thoughts & emotions accompanying it. Interestingly, he points out, this mindfulness training first developed within several religious traditions. We need to learn how to untangle pain: untangle the *sensation* of pain, from our *emotional* response and *imagination*.

Allow me to share an example of **untangling pain**. A long time ago, in a faraway place, I needed a cap placed on a tooth. The dentist numbed my mouth and stepped out for a moment. The receptionist came in and told me the procedure would cost $1000.00. This came as a surprise, as I thought I had insurance; turns out, I exhausted the benefit. I was already numbed and went on with the procedure. Two days later, the tooth was hurting even worse and I needed a root canal, which set me back another $1000.00. As I drove home from the endodontist, I was still in **pain,** and **upset** with the original dentist, for not being upfront about the cost. Only making things worse, I started **imagining** the tooth may need pulled. All the while, ibuprofen was upsetting my stomach and not lasting the full 8 hours. I was not only in pain, but also, suffering as my emotions and imagination were making things worse.

I couldn't sleep, the night after the root canal, so I got up and wrote everything down – I untangled the suffering. I discovered my sensation of pain was entangled in emotion and imagination. I had the toothache, but also, upset with the original dentist (the emotion of anger); all this entangled in imagination, fearing I might need the tooth pulled (which I never did). Now, understanding the predicament, I decided to move on; forgive the dentist and stop pretending I would need the tooth pulled. Finally, having cleared my mind of the **excess baggage**, I was able to concentrate on the pain itself. Since Ibuprofen 800mg was upsetting my stomach, I tried just 400mg; therefore, I could take it every 4 hours, which worked great!

The above example, demonstrates how pain can become entangled in emotion and imagination, resulting in suffering. The untangling process was accomplished using the phenomena, we reviewed in previous chapters, called metacognition (meta meaning "beyond" & cognition meaning "thinking"). Metacognition, thinking about your thinking, occurs in the pre-frontal part of the brain; giving us another way to reduce pain naturally. Mental illness, and improper use of medications, however, can interfere with our metacognitive abilities. Also, our metacognitive abilities need sharpened and prepared for the task, by the honing effect of the spiritual disciplines, we'll review below.

UNDERSTANDING PAIN AND **CORRECT THINKING**

Now that we've looked at the physiological components of pain, let's turn our attention to the cognitive processes of suffering. In the last chapter, we saw how **reductionism** (reducing thinking to brain chemistry) tends to undermine the mental and spiritual aspects of healing. In the same way, we need to distinguish between the biochemical aspects of pain and the metacognitive, mental, and spiritual, aspects of suffering.

The American Medical Association has a pain management program which reviews the "Three Hierarchical Levels of Pain." First, pain has a "sensory discriminative component" (what you actually feel – pains location, intensity, and quality). Pain also has a "motivation-affective component" (influenced by emotions, depression, and anxiety); and finally, a higher "cognitive evaluation component" (our thoughts concerning the cause and significance of the pain). We'll be addressing each of these pain levels as we learn to, **reduce the excess baggage to stay above the "plane of pain."**

These three levels, of course, are not always well defined as we experience pain and suffering. The cingulate cortex, for example, is an area of the brain where thoughts and emotions merge and responds both to physical and emotional pain. **This is important, because, your emotional state definitely influences pain**. Severe emotional arousal increases pain, especially when emotions over-stimulate the autonomic fight or flight and hormonal systems: when your emotions are constantly telling you, something is wrong!

In the last chapter, we saw how things you think about can actually change your brain chemistry. You'll, also recall the Heart Association researchers, showed "changing how an individual thinks about themselves" influenced their ability to change. Correct thinking is the answer to the human condition and becomes very evident in the prevention and treatment of pain. Albert Bandura et al., (1987), did research showing the profound influence thinking can have on pain sensitivity, what he called "cognitive coping." He showed how certain types of thinking, which increases your **self-efficacy**, releases natural opiates into the brain reducing pain; which begs the question, "what is the best type of thinking to improve self-efficacy and reduce pain"?

Correct thinking not only increases our natural pain killers, but also, prevents painful situations. Correct thinking keeps pain in perspective while we experience it. Correct thinking prevents inappropriate use of medications, which, as I've shown, can sometimes worsen pain. Sadly, a major obstacle to correct thinking, is often the pills we use for pain, as drugs can often interfere with optimal brain function. You need to think correctly for metacognition to develop. However, medications can sometimes mess-up your thinking.

Thinking can certainly modify our experience of pain, for better or worse. Pain is increased when it's **unexplained** (Williams & Thorn, 1989). Even the **expectation of pain** causes the release of cholecystokinin (CCK), a chemical which increases pain (Atlas & Wager, 2012). **Our beliefs** can influence pain (Walsh & Radcliff, 2002). Our **prior experiences** with pain can make us more capable of handling it (Höfle, et al., 2012). If we've had experiences with pain and overcame it, we develop performance mastery, which increases our **self-efficacy** and decreases pain (O'Leary, 1985). Albert Bandura showed even a perceived increase in self-efficacy is associated with an increased amount of natural opioid, pain killing, endorphins. However, the moment we take a pill, self-efficacy is reduced, as we come to rely on the medication; therefore, losing our natural abilities. Later, in this chapter, we'll look at cognitive coping techniques which will increase your self-efficacy, and along with that, your natural ability to both withstand and reduce pain.

There's a well-known correlation between chronic pain, mental illness, and medication overuse. Once again we can find individuals trapped in the middle of a vicious cycle.

TRAPPED

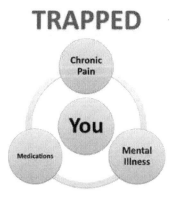

Chronic pain is often treated with medications, and yet, medications can sometimes cause chronic pain. Medications, used to treat mental illness, can sometimes lead to depression and anxiety. Finally, mental illness can heighten pain perception, which often increases depression and anxiety. The individual is stuck in the middle of a triangle: trapped in pain, mental illness, and often taking medications which are no longer helping, and even, making things worse. Addictionologist's often talk about the downward spiral, which destroys a life, when opioids and benzodiazepines (antianxiety mediations) are used together.[8]

There's a significant association between chronic nonmalignant pain and mental illness. 65% of chronic pain patients have at least one psychiatric disorder and 56% have a major depressive disorder (Dersh et al., 2006). Likewise, "On average, 65% of patients with depression experience one or more pain complaints" (Bair et al., 2003). Pain psychiatrist, Patrick Gibbons, suggests many stressed-out people tend to focus their stress into a bodily ailment (Gibbons, 2009). But, often simply identifying the emotional response to the stress, will improve the painful situation. Gibbons talks about a

---

[8] Benzodiazepines are drugs such as lorazepam (Ativan), alprazolam (Xanax), diazepam (Valium), and clonazepam (Klonopin).

condition called 'alexithymia' where people have trouble identifying and expressing emotions, and therefore, tend to experience emotional stress as physical pain.

"Chronic Pain Syndrome" is the name given to chronic pain associated with mental illness; defined as, "pain greater than 3 months, anxiety or depression and loss of function." It's important to distinguish chronic pain from chronic pain syndrome, as the latter can be significantly improved by correct thinking; and yet, our medical community often feeds us pills and lies rather than correct thinking! Dr. Miriam Grossman, a college campus psychiatrist, rocked the world of traditional psychiatry in 2006. Her book, *Unprotected (a campus psychiatrist reveals how political correctness in her profession endangers every student),* was originally authored as 'Anonymous M.D.' due to the truthfulness of her claims. Dr. Grossman exposes our healthcare system as suffering from Theophobia (having an irrational fear of God). "How scandalous, that the very profession we trust to guide and heal is sowing confusion and illness." She goes on to discuss the field of "Neurotheology."

Healthcare providers need to get over their theophobia and understand the importance of nurturing our spirit; developing the "platform" we sit on to look back upon ourselves, allowing us to rise above ourselves, and identify thought processes and emotions that maybe contributing to pain. **Spiritual development helps us stay above the 'plane of pain' by a process known as cognitive restructuring**. Viktor Frankl said, "Emotion, which is suffering, ceases to be suffering as soon as we form a clear and precise picture of it." Spiritual development gives us the ability to paint a clear picture of pain. Learning to control our big human brain is so important; spirituality assists us in the process.

OVERCOMING PAIN

Spirituality gives us another instrument in our tool shed; rather than, just scalpels & pills, or what Dr. Gibbons called "**chemical coping**"! God thinking, in particular, the type of God thinking Christianity produces, sets in motion a series of thinking (cognitive) events, healing us mentally and physically. However, the tool of spirituality, as suggested in the last chapter, needs to be developed because it lacks structure; the structure, Jesus's teaching on the Kingdom of God provides.

Skeptical? Let's put it to the test and investigate how to control pain by applying spiritual concepts. Albert Bandura showed the profound influence self-efficacy and proper thinking can have on the level of our natural painkillers – "**cognitive coping**." Dr. Esmer reported on the effects of "Mindfulness Based" pain control. Dr. Schubiner talks about the "Mind Body Syndrome": how the mind can twist the body into pain. The larger question becomes, what kind of thinking best improves our self-efficacy, and along with it, our natural pain killing abilities; what kind of thinking best enhances our mindfulness; what kind of thinking best gets us to a higher level or plane, to untangle and untwist a chronic painful experience? Jesus' teaching on the Kingdom of God best fulfills all the requirements!

I've defined five characteristics of Kingdom walkers, five ways to increase your self-efficacy: **understanding, joy, prayer, trust, and hope**. With all due respect, these five characteristics best develop the self-efficacy Bandura was looking for; increases mindfulness better than Esmer's mindfulness training; and, as Schubiner was looking for, best untangles a body twisted into pain!

Understanding

Pain is such an overwhelming sensation we often just experience it, as it **overcomes us**! It's easy to get lost in the experience of pain, saying, "I hate this, life is awful, why would God allow something so terrible." This kind of response is normal and natural; however, it is just a "knee jerk" response to a bad situation. Like all situations in life we need to apply understanding. Letting our emotions take over and getting mad at God, only makes things worse. Recall the American Medical Associations, pain management series, refers to the "cognitive evaluation component" (our thoughts concerning the cause and significance of the pain). Our thoughts about pain itself, why God would even allow such a thing, cannot be neglected. To ignore our thoughts is to ignore the development and nurturing of humanities greatest ability!

When painful circumstances arise, we need to step back, onto our spirit, and look at them in the total context of life; understanding Gods love and ability to care for His children. When we apply understanding to experience, suffering seems to dissipate. Also, Christianity gives us the best worldview to understand suffering. If we have no overall worldview, suffering seems meaningless, and the meaninglessness, only makes the suffering worse.

C.S. Lewis did a wonderful job applying understanding to pain in his book *The Problem of Pain* (1940). Lewis teaches us to apply understanding to painful situations, so, we can move beyond the "unthinking" response: I'll share some of his thoughts with you below. When we suffer, in our emotional distress, we tend to doubt God's **goodness and love, but also, His greatness and fairness**.

The Veracity of God

To understand how God could allow pain and suffering; which, helps our <u>cognitive evaluation</u> of pain, we need to understand Gods character. God's goodness consists of moral purity, love, and integrity. Integrity involves three things: genuineness (being true), **veracity** (telling the truth) and faithfulness (proves true). When God created life, He didn't lie to us, or hide, the existence of evil; He's going to display veracity and tell the truth. However, even with his veracity, we know His overall integrity stands true: He's also faithful, loving, and pure.

The presence of evil, and experience of pain, also calls into question God's attributes of goodness and greatness: either God is not totally good, or, He's not totally God, and in control. This problem, by the way, is not unique to Christianity; all world religions must come up with a theodicy. Theodicy refers to man's attempts to justify the ways of God. A theodicy is proving God right even in a very wrong world. Theodicy answers the question, "why does God allow pain and evil to exist." First, we'll look at Gods **goodness,** then His **greatness**; but, in the end, we must humble ourselves and remember a simple childhood prayer, "God is good, God is great, thank-you for this food, Amen." Sometimes it's enough just knowing who God is and being thankful for all we have.

God is Good

We're created in God's image and **He's given us his name!** God has many names reflecting his numerous characteristics. Conner & Malmin, in their book, *The Covenants, The Key to God's Relationship with Mankind* (1983), suggests the ultimate triune name of God. The name which reflects the trinity and God's final "Everlasting Covenant" with man, is the name "LORD JESUS CHRIST." The people of God, they tell us, often became **partakers of the name** of God, with whom they were in covenantal relationship: "Because the believer in Christ is under the New Covenant, he also is in covenantal relationship with God through Christ, by the Spirit, and thus partakers of the triune covenantal and great redemptive name of the Lord Jesus Christ" (p.110). We're the children, the offspring, of the Most High and Holy God. We are even called by His name! Whether the theologically inclined reader agrees with Conner & Malmin is beside the point. We can all agree, with great **distinction** comes great challenges. The point is, we seriously underestimate our authority and position in the universe, as beings capable of thinking and relating to God, and, all the accompanying responsibility and consequences. **Pain and suffering seems unfair if we underestimate the gift of eternal life in the name of Jesus.**

It comes down to the basics of 'life' itself. Regardless of whether we like it, God created life and said, "It is good." We sometimes may not agree, but, God said, "It is good" and it is good! Even suffering from hunger, Jesus said, "Is not **life** more important than food." Jesus had a much higher view of life than the apparent quality of it at any particular time (see appendix 1, The Numinous). Life itself, the simple fact of life, is good and more important than uncomfortable and even painful circumstances.

God is Great

Pain, suffering, and evil often seem unchecked: it's natural to wonder "who's in charge here." Pain calls God's omnipotence into question. God is good, but, maybe He's not totally in control. C. S. Lewis (1940, p.18) suggests two things must be present for human life to exist: freewill and an 'inexorable nature."

To understand man's **freewill,** it's important to realize God cannot actualize a contradiction. Lewis writes, "if you choose to say 'God can give a creature free will and at the same time withhold free will from it', you have not succeeded in saying anything about God." Either God gave us freewill or he didn't. Mankind's freedom, as opposed to God sovereignty, is debated throughout the ages. To answer this seeming contradiction Hoekema (1994) presents the idea of "**created persons**." We are "**created**" beings, ultimately under the control of a sovereign God. He also created us as "**persons**" suggesting a degree of personal freedom. Which type of God is greater: A God who can work the universe like a puppet, or, a greater God, who can allow man certain freedoms, with all it fearsomeness, and still fulfill His ultimate will (source unknown)? Man's freewill doesn't reduce God's control and greatness, but, does introduce the possibility of pain and evil. So, the question, Lewis asks, asked "are we suffering too much pain or too much freedom"?

The second essential characteristic for human life to exist, according to Lewis, is an '**inexorable nature**'. The laws of nature cannot be moved.

> The inexorable 'laws of Nature' which operate in
> defiance of human suffering or desert, which are not
> turned aside by prayer, seem, at first sight, to furnish
> a strong argument against the goodness and power of
> God. I am going to submit that not even
> Omnipotence could create a society of free souls
> without at the same time creating a relatively
> independent and 'inexorable' Nature (Ibid, p.19).

For mankind to exist there must be some laws of nature we can count on, even if these laws, sometimes, hurt. God cannot actualize a contradiction: He cannot make a round square. God cannot make human beings in His image, able to think and have certain freedoms, and suddenly, take freedom away. God cannot create laws of nature, and then, suddenly allow them to be broken. God created laws of nature and freewill creatures; sometimes, they interact in ways uncomfortable for us.

God and man have freedoms; but, God's freedom looks somewhat different than man's. Lewis goes on to explain,

> The freedom of God consists in the fact that no cause
> other than Himself produces His acts and no external
> obstacle impedes them – that his own goodness is the
> root from which they (His acts) all grow and his own
> omnipotence the air in which they (again His acts) all
> flower" (Ibid, p27, parenthesis added).

In talking about God's act's, which includes life: they **must** all originate from God's goodness and **must** be sustained by his greatness! "God is obligated to create the best" (Feinberg, 2005, p.1185).

God is fair and loving

God is good and God is great but does he really love us? Is God fair? The Bible book of *Job* is about pain, suffering, and God's fairness. Many believe *Job* was the first book of the bible ever written; suggesting, God wanted to get this pain situation understood from the very beginning. God does understand our suffering and our need to understand it. Despite all his suffering, Job never calls God's goodness or greatness into question, rather, wonders about His **justice**. Job suggests God may not be fair: the entire book is built around Job asking for his day in court. Once again, we must simply rely on faith. Job 4:17 says, "Shall mortal man be more just than God? shall a man be more pure than his maker." God is good and great, also, a 'just' & loving God. He weeps with those who weep!

Susan, a young girl in C.S Lewis' classic book, *The Lion the Witch and the Wardrobe,* looks toward the godlike lion figure and asks if he is safe. Mr. Beaver responds, "Course he (God) isn't safe. But he's good." They go on to suggest, "He is not a tame Lion." No, God is not tame toward people created in his image, who stand to inherit the glory of His Son!

> You asked for a loving God: you have one. The great spirit you so lightly invoked, the **'lord of terrible aspect'** is present: not a senile benevolence that drowsily wishes you to be happy in your own way, not the cold philanthropy of a conscience magistrate, nor the care of a host who feels responsible for the comfort of his guests, but the consuming fire himself (Lewis, 1940, p.39).

God's goodness cannot be separated from His love! Love is more than kindness, and we are the objects of God's love. Lewis writes, "Whether we like it or not, God intends to give us what we need, not what we now think we want. Once more, we are embarrassed by the intolerable compliment, by too much love, not too little" (Ibid, pp 46-47). The "problem of pain" is only a problem in the eyes of unrepentant men.

We must attend to the <u>cognitive needs</u> of those who are suffering. I'm making the case for understanding and not just experiencing pain. Recall, Emily Dickinson wrote "pain has… no future but itself, Its infinite realms contain Its past, enlightened to perceive new periods of pain." When we're in pain, we really are on a different plane of existence. Therefore, when we must board this "plane of pain" we need to "limit the emotional baggage" and replace it with the "carry on case of understanding." As much as possible, we do need to "keep calm and carry on."

Unfortunately, nothing disrupts our thinking quit like pain. Therefore, our thinking, as much as possible, should take flight above and transcend the experience of pain; even entering the realm of spirit! Recall, I've defined an aspect of spirit as a higher level of thinking, which isn't grounded to just the world around us, or even to our physical state, at the moment. However, this realm of spirituality, this realm of higher thinking, thinking about our thinking, thinking about things we cannot see; what cognitive researchers have defined as metacognition, needs to be developed.

Joy

Joy is the second way to increase self-efficacy; and along with that, your natural pain fighting ability. Kingdom walkers are frequently heard using the word 'joy', best defined as, "A state of delight and **wellbeing** that comes from knowing and serving God" (Dean, 2003, p.956). I like this definition, because it emphasizes a sense of 'well-being'. Illicit drug use is man's desperate and relentless search for this sense of wellbeing and security, which Christians receive naturally as one of the spiritual "fruits" we call joy.

The definition above also emphasizes "delight." The Nucleus Accumbiens is the pleasure and delight center of the brain. Our society has become very adept at overstimulating the Nucleus Accumbiens, using drugs, alcohol, food, gambling, and sex. Even the very thought of these activities activates our pleasure pathways (indicating the power of thought). Once again, the bigger question becomes, what type of thinking, what spirit, most productively and resourcefully activates the Nucleus Accumbiens. Our pleasure center was given to us to be stimulated by <u>natural</u> things, such as controlled eating, marital intercourse, the warm feeling of security we get from shelter, but also, the wellbeing that comes from the worship of God. The bible teaches us to rejoice in the Lord. Yes, 'knowing and serving God' does produce feelings of euphoria. He's our real source of pleasure, security, and wellbeing. To deny this, is to deny yourself an infinite and inexhaustible source of wellbeing! Recall, emotional pain is sometimes misconstrued as physical pain: joy helps to keep us calm, and gives us a sense of security, which also reduces suffering.

Prayer

Prayer is the third, and most important, tool to control pain and suffering. Jesus taught us to use prayer as our primary source of healing and pain relief. **Prayer, being the most effective platform for reflection, gets us away from ourselves**. Ketamine, an anesthetic drug sometimes used during surgery, is considered a dissociative anesthetic: dissociating the conscious mind from other parts of the brain. Ketamine helps relieve pain by dissociating mind from body; producing dream-like states, trances, and euphoria. Opioids and other drugs, including marijuana, have some dissociative properties, as they help people "get away from themselves." Prayer could be considered a natural dissociative agent! Psychiatrist, Dr. Miriam Grossman (2006) points to research on prayer:

> They scanned the heads of skilled Tibetan meditators
> and Franciscan nuns following a period of intense

religious contemplation and discovered an unusual pattern of brain activity. As peak moments approached, the circuits responsible for orientation in time and space fell quiet. The area of the brain that informs us where we end, and the rest of the world starts, was turned off. These moments, according to the subjects, were accompanied by a rush of positive emotion. They were moments of 'being connected to all creation,' of 'a sense of timelessness and infinity' and 'a tangible sense of the closeness of God and a mingling with Him'.

These Tibetan monks and Franciscan nuns could break the boundaries of self, time, and space by prayer. Nothing separates us from the world, and develops our spirit, like prayer!

What I mean by prayer and what many others experience, are usually two different things. Prayer is a purposefully arranged meeting, where a discussion is held with the founder and sustainer of the universe! Historically, Christians have held to a "sweet hour of prayer," as Jesus lamented in the Garden of Gethsemane, that his disciples couldn't stay awake with Him even for an hour. As Dr. Esmer, develops his "mindfulness" approach to natural pain relief he encourages his pain patients to meditate 45 minutes a day. How important is controlling pain? Do you want it bad enough to purposefully develop a prayer life? Do you want it bad enough to pray an hour every day?

People often talk about going into a prayer closet which can be confusing. No one is suggesting prayer be confined to a closet; I would suggest, however, a dedicated space, which over time develops into a sanctuary separated from the rest of the world. I heard Dr. David Jeramiah talk about kneeling in prayer, but, often found himself "resting in the Lord" (asleep). During my prayer time, I may be found kneeling, sitting in a chair, sometimes flat on my face before my Maker, most often, pacing and talking aloud, doing business with God! Regardless of the prayer posture, a sense of timelessness and connectedness to God develops, even as a separation from this world occurs. Life itself is given to us, to develop prayer and spend time with God!

Trust

Trust is the fourth characteristic Jesus taught us, which increases self-efficacy and reduces pain. Luke 18:17 says, "Truly I say to you, whoever does not receive the kingdom of God like a child shall not enter it at all." We must, not only have trust and faith, but possess **childlike** trust and faith. We trust our King: knowing He cares for us and understands the pain we endure – and has a plan for all this!

Hope

Finally, Jesus taught us the importance of hope! The heartbeat of the Kingdom of God is the heartbeat of eternity. Kingdom walkers always have an eternal perspective and a tight hold on the "rope of hope" firmly secured in the true tabernacle of God, in the true eternal Kingdom! We must always apply hope to any painful situation. Romans 8:26 tells us hope is the means, through which, the Holy Spirit heals us. Healing is uniquely extended as we hope! However, "chronic pain", by definition, is loss of hope.

When we're ill, in pain, or suffering in some way, our first response should always be to look to the Lord and have faith He can heal us. We need to hope in God first for our healing, to His *special grace*, and then to the *common grace* of our healthcare systems. Even if God chooses not to heal us immediately, we can always find comfort in Him. Romans 8 goes on and tells us, "all things", even suffering, "works together for good to those who love God, to those who are called according to His purpose." Psychologist and Pastor J. E. Rose looks at hope as a neural model, its purpose is to fill in the gaps of our knowledge and to supply meaning to the events in our lives. Hope fills in the gaps when we don't understand suffering.

making it more tolerable!

PLANTED FOR SUCCESS

Correct thinking reduces the sensation of pain, by increasing our body's natural pain killers; but also, correct thinking helps control emotions & stress, which reduces the experience of suffering! **Understanding, joy, prayer, trust and hope** are particularly well suited to fulfill any of the criteria developed by Bandura, Esmer or Schubiner. These five characteristics are best cultivated in the setting of a church; together, with other Christian people. I love the analogy of the church being like a campfire. One log by itself cannot sustain a fire, it takes several together. Also, baptism usually occurs in the setting of a church. Baptism "unites" us with Jesus, giving us strength to overcome old, destructive, and painful habits. I've discussed the birth of our new spirit, the process of being born again: baptism "plants us for success"!

I've got **Good News**! You can overcome possession by pain and pills. Your life can be renewed! Baptism is an amazing and mystical experience. Being immersed in baptismal water "plants" us with Jesus.[9] Then, like a flower growing from a planted seed, we're raised, out of the water with Christ, "to walk in newness of life"! Now is the time for your baptism. Even now, call a trusted spiritual leader and tell him/her you're ready to be healed of pain; you're ready to be baptized; you're ready to be "planted for success"!

MOVING FROM PRINCIPLE TO PRAXIS

The ability to move from principle to praxis, taking theory with us into action, becomes urgent as we board the plane of pain. Pain often presents itself as a "disorienting dilemma": pain knocks us off

---

[9] Rom 6:5 KJV - For if we have been **planted** together in the likeness of his death, we shall be also [in the likeness] of [his] resurrection

our feet! Disorienting dilemmas, however, are part of the Transformational Learning process. Disorienting dilemmas, like pain, catalyze perspective transformation, which can result in sudden dramatic lifestyle changes! Disorienting dilemmas according to M. Carolyn Clark (1993),

> present a serious challenge to life as the person has known it…it presents a threat or rupture of the person's life fabric…disorienting dilemma demands some immediate action from the person. Thrown off balance, they must do something to regain equilibrium; and since the old ways have been challenged, this means trying something radically new.

Indeed, something radically new is required, as current ways of dealing with chronic pain are failing. Turk et al., (2011), after reviewing all **conventional** treatments modalities available for chronic nonmalignant pain wrote, "the best evidence for pain reduction averages roughly 30% in about half of treated patients, and these pain reductions do not always occur with concurrent improvement in function." Clearly a different, **holistic**, approach to pain is necessary.

Just as we used depression for case study in *Understanding Mental Health,* we're going to use knee osteoarthritis as an example in *Overcoming Pain.* "Knee osteoarthritis is the most frequent cause of mobility dependency and diminished quality of life" in the United States (Messier, 2013). Knee replacements are expected to increase 673% by 2030 (Kurtz, 2007). The results of sawing through bones and screwing in new joints can be painful. The real suffering, however, occurred in the years leading up to the joint replacement. Osteoarthritis, often erroneously termed 'wear and tear' arthritis, is epidemic in our country and provides a good case study for the application of the holistic concepts we've developed.

The common "wear & tear" fallacy can result in compliancy as the individual believes the disease is inevitable and nothing can be done. Again, we see how beliefs bubble out into behavior. However, Dr. Greg Wade (2011) challenges the conventional understanding of osteoarthritis, as an inevitable disease of aging, suggesting it's "the result of a definable history in the individual." Arthritis, like many chronic pain syndromes, is often the result of individual lifestyle choices. Lifestyle changes can be intimidating; however, the concepts we've developed can maximize your success in reducing pain, allowing you to prevent disease and age gracefully. The previous chapters laid the spiritual scaffolding needed to enter a discussion of diet, weight control and exercise without the fear of failure. Therefore, with the above concepts in mind, we'll review how the pain and loss of function associated with osteoarthritis, and other chronic painful conditions, can be prevented and, in many cases, even reversed.

The University of Michigan once had a billboard that read "Knowledge is Healing." That's so true! Data from the Health and Retirement Study showed the "better-educated are better able to manage chronic conditions and have better health outcomes" (Margolis, 2013). Therefore, let's review two landmark studies concerning lifestyle issues and pain.

McCarthy et.al., (2009) looked at results from the Einstein Aging Study and discovered a correlation between chronic pain and obesity in the elderly: "obese subjects were twice as likely and severely obese subjects were more than four times as likely as normal weighted subjects to have chronic pain." In addition to the increased mechanical load across weight bearing joints, they also found "obesity is a pro-inflammatory state", associated with higher pain causing chemicals in the body. "Obese subjects were significantly more likely to have chronic pain in the head, neck or shoulder, back, legs or feet, and abdomen or pelvis than subjects who were not obese."

Researchers from Wake Forest University looked at the effects of intensive diet and exercise on knee joints loads and inflammation (Messier et al., 2013). They discovered these obesity related inflammatory chemicals diffused into the joint lining and muscles causing pain. This definitive study compared the effects on exercise alone, diet alone and finally diet and exercise together. They found weight change not only reduced knee compression forces, but also, reduced pain chemicals in joint fluid, resulting in significantly improved pain and function scores, in just 18 months. Of course, the diet and exercise groups did better than either group alone.

Clearly diet and exercise are necessary to prevent and treat arthritis, and other pain syndromes; but, stretching is also very important. Patients sometimes present with knee pain even after a joint replacement. Usually, the cause of the pain is same thing which led to the arthritis in the first place: weak muscles along with tight ligaments and tendons across the joint. The new knee didn't fix these soft tissue problems. Likewise, studies have shown joint pain after activity is usually not from the joint itself, but structures around the joint – such as muscles, ligaments, and tendons. Stretching can free up limited joint mobility, reduce the risk of arthritis, and reduce pain. Stretching is the fountain of youth!

Osteoarthritis is characterized by joint stiffness; however, Dr. Wade suggests "joint restriction is causal rather than symptomatic": it's not the arthritis that restricted moment, but rather, the restricted movement caused the arthritis. Preventing joint stiffness with stretching is essential to good health and joint protection. Stretching helps prevent and treat arthritis by keeping the ligaments across the joints freed up, thus reducing abnormal wear patterns; it's important to make sure the joints stay stretched out so they can move freely. Wade suggests "preserving joint mobility offers the possibility of arresting further (joint) degeneration" and "self-management with stretching is effective in indefinitely prolonging treatment efficacy." Stretching also releases endorphins, natural pain killers, into body tissues.

To prevent pain and stiffness, joints should be used, remain freed-up and mobile, through stretching and strengthening. However, the position of the joint is also important. There's fibrous tissue around joints, called the joint capsule. When the joint is straight, the capsule is opened-up into a relaxed position. However, when joints are bent, as found in a seated position, there is "maximum capsular torsion"; the joint capsule is pulled tight, placing abnormal pressure points on the cartilage. Prolonged compression, from sitting too much, can actually wear on the joint! We need to stand more and sit less!

Moderate strength training also stabilizes and protects joints by preventing abnormal movements. One study showed a 53% reduction in pain associated with rheumatoid arthritis after just 16 weeks of strength training (Flint-Wagner et al., 2009). Also, joints which are properly stretched and strengthened heal quicker and less likely to be injured.

The problem is aerobic exercise, strength training and even stretching can be painful, especially to already arthritic joints. However, we have to get away from the mindset that all pain is evil and must be avoided at all costs. **Kinesiophobia** is an irrational fear of movement; believing we should never do anything which hurts. This fear of movement can get blown out of proportion (catastrophized) and can even lead to worsening pain intensity. Keep in mind, **"muscles and joints that don't move hurt."**

Sometimes the best thing for a painful joint, muscle or tendon is to massage, move and gently stretch it! Massage and mobility can help the healing process and stimulate natural pain killers in the tissues. If your endorphins, natural painkillers, are already built up from exercise, you can even get a sense of relief or pleasure from rubbing, moving, or gently stretching a painful condition. Of course, I'm not referring to an acute severe injury, like a broken bone. C.S. Lewis (1940) suggests, "If I trust my own feeling, a slight aching in the legs as we climb into bed after a good day's walking is, in fact, pleasurable." Lewis can say this because walking has generated natural opioids in his system to combat the aching pain from the walk!

CONCLUSION

Abraham Maslow's *Law of the Instrument* says, "If the only tool you have is a hammer every problem looks like a nail." If the only tool we have to treat pain is a pill, well then, the "god-almighty" pill is the best tool for the job! If the only tools we have are owned by orthopedic surgeons, then, surgery is the answer. My goal, in this chapter, was to give you tools to manage pain, prevent dependency, and increase self-efficacy. I gave you the tool of understanding: understanding pain and pain pathways, and how we can manipulate these pain pathways, in natural ways. I showed how the tools of exercise and stretching can be used to prevent and manage the pain of chronic arthritis and other conditions.

Drug rehabilitation programs often see chronic pain improve when opiates are discontinued. Medications can sometimes interfere with our God given way of dealing with pain. Opioids, nerve pills, certain types of muscle relaxers, and sleep aids, can result in **cognitive** (thinking) **impairment**. I've discussed how important thinking is to untangle pain. Unfortunately, medications can sometimes cloud your thinking, and even result in depressed mood, which can all worsen internal pain perception.

Don J. Kurth M.D. (2006), former Medical Director of the Chemical Dependency Center at Loma Linda University, suggested "Opioid therapy can lead to **spiritual death**"! Our brain must function properly to understand reality, God, and His plan for our lives. The New Testament, Greek word, for magic arts and witchcraft is **pharmakia,** from which we get our word 'pharmacy'. Many assume, as long as their physician prescribes the medication, it must be ok. This cannot be further from the truth. When we rely **solely** on pills for relief of life's problems we're really just practicing modern day witchcraft, which God abhors. The very last chapter of the bible tells us sorcerers, those who practice pharmakia, will not enter the Kingdom of God!

CHAPTER 5

DISEASE PREVENTION AND LIFESTYLE

In the first century Jesus walked the earth healing people but in the 21st century He's given us knowledge to prevent disease!

Our goal in this chapter is to make real and lasting lifestyle modifications allowing us to go from healthcare to self-care. The previous chapters were designed to get us to the point where disease prevention is even possible; and, as we look ahead, graceful aging is impossible without prevention. We've looked at your ability to change and the concept of a transformational journey. This chapter will move forward and suggest a continuing process of **lifestyle upgrades.** However, the profound lifestyle changes I'm suggesting requires a holistic approach, allowing God to show us the "path of life." Few spiritual leaders have entered into the arena of healthcare and made as great an impact as Ellen White. As we go along, I would like to share a few quotes from Ellen: "Pure air, sunlight, abstemiousness, rest, exercise, proper diet, the use of water, trust in divine power—these are the true remedies.... Health does not depend on chance" (White, 2004, p290).

A core principle of adult learning (andragogy) suggests "Adults need to know why they need to learn something before learning it" (Holton, 2001). It's sometimes hard to follow rules and make changes if someone gives suggestions without explanations. Knowledge and skills are much easier to masticate if we understand why we need to digest it, and not just have it "shoved down our throats." If we understand the reason behind the suggestion, motivation often comes naturally, so it is with our health. If I can show you why exercise, diet and weight control are so important, and then, lead you in a process of gradual transformation, you'll be much more likely to establish lasting lifestyle changes. First we'll look at diet, then exercise, and finally, learn how to apply the principles we've learned (moving from principle to praxis)

DIET

"As a strong wind sweeps away a boat on the water, even one of the roaming senses on which the mind focuses can carry away a man's intelligence" Swami Prabhupada

The National Opinion Research Center (Tompson, et al., 2012) looked into our level of health understanding as they polled over a 1000 people. 78% knew being overweight leads to heart disease, and 70% knew it caused diabetes, but only 7% knew being overweight could cause cancer. However, "One-third of the cancer deaths that occur each year can be attributed to diet and physical activity" (Wiseman, 2008). This finding is staggering! Think about the suffering from even one case of cancer: the shock of finding out you or a loved one has cancer; all the testing, surgery, radiation, and effects of chemotherapy, not to mention possibly dying, from even one case of cancer. Now image all the suffering in the world related to cancer. Finally, imagine removing 1/3 of all that suffering, just by eating right and exercising. They said we can remove another one third by getting rid of tobacco. So two-thirds of all cancer is lifestyle related! There's no doubt diet has influenced the epidemic of cancer.

Researchers from Kaiser Permanente followed 6,500 people for 36 years, and reported in the Journal of Neurology, that central obesity gives us a threefold increased risk of dementia (Whitmer, et al., 2008). The Journal of the American Medical Association (JAMA) reported August 2009, "The Mediterranean diet may have a beneficial effect during the prodromal phase of dementia" (Féart, et al., 2009). Although diet will not reverse the effects of dementia, they suggest the Mediterranean diet may help slow its development.

Preventing cancer and dementia is important; however, the

biggest killer in our country is hardening of the arteries or atherosclerosis, leading to heart attacks, strokes, amputations, and some types of dementia. Although family history plays a part, diet and exercise are necessary for disease prevention. Thankfully, **very simple** changes in our lifestyle can make a big difference! I've seen people lose tremendous amounts of weight by understanding just a few important dietary principles. Therefore, let's look at "Syndrome X."

Elevated cholesterol, diabetes and high blood pressure seemed epidemic in our country; the combination of these conditions was originally named Syndrome X. Ultimately, the common underlying cause is actually too much **insulin**. This is important to understand because **foods which increase insulin are deadly!** I want you to understand how to avoid high insulin levels which ultimately leads to high blood pressure, cholesterol, obesity and, contrary to what you may think, high insulin can actually cause type 2 diabetes.

Before I explain insulin resistance, as you know, there are a lot of questionable teachings in the world, especially in relation to diet, this is not one of them! What I'm about to tell you is science, its reality, and understanding this material is going to help you lose weight and maintain a healthy weight. Understanding this material will help put pieces of the dietary puzzle together, help you make better food choices, upgrade your diet, and the pounds will fall off!

As you know, sugar turns on insulin production. Insulin is a hormonal key which moves sugar from blood into cells. If you have too many insulin keys, the locks become dysfunctional (resistant to the effects of insulin) and **insulin resistance** develops. It's important to understand that abdominal fat turns on insulin production much like eating sugar. There's more blood supply in your abdomen than anywhere else in your body, so abdominal 'free fatty acids' are continuously delivered, 24 hours a day, into the blood stream resulting in dangerously high insulin levels.

Understanding insulin resistance is very important! If the body is resistant to insulin (because of central obesity) then blood sugar slowly increases, which increases insulin levels even more, resulting in a vicious cycle.

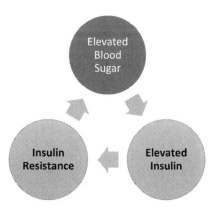

Insulin resistance is the cause of adult onset (type 2 diabetes). If the body is resistant to the effects of insulin then blood sugar slowly increases, resulting in even higher insulin and more resistance (more insulin "lock" dysfunction). Thus a vicious cycle develops: too much sugar leading to too much insulin, insulin resistance leading back to elevated sugar, and the cycle goes on. Now, with that understood, we can lay the final piece of the puzzle, leading to your first heart attack!

High insulin, from central obesity and increased sugar intake, causes blood pressure to increase. This high insulin also causes bad LDL cholesterol and triglycerides to go up, and this high insulin causes protective HDL cholesterol to go down. Finally, the important **take home message**, and the reason we've reviewed all this, **insulin makes you hungry**, further increasing your weight. So an even a bigger vicious cycle develops: too much weight leading to **elevated insulin** levels, insulin makes us **hungry** so we **eat more** which causes increasing **central obesity** and the cycle continues on. Now that we understand insulin metabolism the name Syndrome X has been replaced by "Metabolic Syndrome."

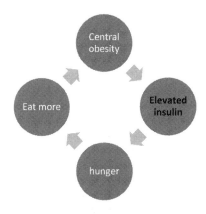

If you're struggling with weight and hungry all the time, you probably have elevated insulin levels fueling the gears of two vicious cycles leading to poor health. One cycle inside your body, biochemically, with elevated insulin leading to receptor "lock" dysfunction and insulin resistance, leading to elevated blood sugar. But also, outside the biochemical level, we see another cycle in our day to day life; elevated insulin causing us to feel hungry all the time, leading to central obesity, and resulting increased fat in the blood, which further increases insulin.

In summary: ELEVATED INSULIN (FROM BEING OVERWEIGHT) INCREASES BLOOD PRESSURE AND CHOLESTEROL AND, BECAUSE OF INSULIN RESISTANCE, WE DEVELOP DIABETES. TOGETHER THESE RISKS ULTIMATELY CAUSE HARDING OF THE ARTERIES WHICH LEADS TO STROKES, HEART ATTACKS AND EVEN DEMENTIA!

Another trap has developed. We saw a trap in mental illness, a trap in chronic pain, and now I've exposed a physical, metabolic trap in our bodies! So what's the way out? We've spent a lot of time on this because understanding insulin resistance allows you to make better food choices. We need to avoid food and beverages which increase insulin production. Also, because elevated insulin makes us hungry, it's hard to start dieting; however, after just a couple of days of appropriate food intake, your insulin levels will come down and dieting will become easier. Of course, many people are **prescribed** insulin and dependent on it for their **lives**, which is a totally different situation. If you've been prescribed insulin, don't stop it unless directed by your healthcare provider.

Before we move on, one final summary is appropriate. Being overweight causes too much insulin. Insulin makes you hungry which further increases weight. Insulin increases blood pressure and cholesterol, leading to heart disease and stroke. That's metabolic syndrome. But I've also heard this referred to as "C.H.A.O.S.", an acronym for Coronary artery disease, Hypertension, Adult onset diabetes, Obesity, and Stroke. We tend to give names to bad situations then walk away unmoved. The things we're reviewing are very real and very serious; I'm talking about CHAOS, a storm that suddenly moves in and destroys your life.

Your living your normal life and then comes this crushing chest pressure, you can't breathe and think maybe your dying; this is different from other experiences with panic and fear, because you are dying, you're having a "coronary", a heart attack, and soon in an ambulance on your way to the emergency room, wondering how all this will turn out. At the very least you're going to get a heart catheterization but maybe a bypass, if you live. What about a stroke? Again, living your normal life, but now do it without speaking or using your right arm. Researchers are also considering the links between insulin resistance & some forms of breast, prostate, and colon cancer. We've already reviewed how elevated insulin can lead to depression, but also, to chronic pain; all because of sugar and insulin metabolism.

Avoid Foods Which Turn on Insulin

What can be done to turn down insulin levels? Sometimes very simple changes in diet can make weight fall off easily! Just remember the principle of avoiding insulin production. The first thing to eliminate is **liquid calories**, as they're absorbed very quickly from the stomach, into the blood stream, demanding immediate and high insulin production. Even "good" drinks such as orange juice and milk are loaded with these "bio-available" calories. Sugar sweetened beverages, like pop and tea, but also, juices and milk, must be eliminated completely from your diet or you will not lose weight!

Let's quickly compare drinking orange juice vs. eating the orange: same amount of fruit sugar but orange juice sugar is absorbed very fast from the stomach, turning on high insulin production (making you hungry and turning fruit sugar into fat); whereas, the pulp and fiber in the orange, as grown, slows the absorption of the sugar, sneaking by the pancreas without releasing so much insulin. Researchers are also discovering something in the way fruits, as grown, are structured that reduces the fruit sugars contact with the absorptive surface of the intestinal wall.

You've arrived at a very important juncture in your life. If you're serious about achieving and maintaining lean body weight something must change! I'll be making a lot of suggestions, and you can dismiss them all, leading to dependency on your doctor and the healthcare system or commit to something and change. I can't emphasis this enough, DO NOT DRINK ANYTHING WITH CALORIES IN IT! It's not just liquid calories that turn on insulin but also **refined simple sugars**, such as ice cream, donuts, cakes, cookies, and candies. These are wasted calories and as we age our body requires less and less calories; thus, learning to break the addiction to sugar is important.

Sugars also appear in other deadly forms: breads and pastas. These starches are simply sugar molecules all stuck together. As we sit down to a bowl of spaghetti we're really sitting down to a bowl of sugar – that's all it is! These foods are not absorbed quickly into the circulation, like simple sugars, but are steadily absorbed keeping insulin levels high for hours. As you know sugars are carbohydrates, one of the three major food groups and the body's main source of energy. But, we need to choose our carbohydrates wisely. We need to choose God made carbs over man made carbs. Carbohydrates found in fruits, vegetables and legumes should make up the largest percentage of our daily caloric intake.

Sugar not only turns on insulin, resulting in insulin resistance; sugar also turns on **genes** that make you fat! The New England Journal of Medicine suggested sugar sweetened beverages may actually turn on genes for obesity. "The genetic association with adiposity appeared to be more pronounced with the greater intake of sugar-sweetened beverages" (Qi, et.al., 2012). We all know obesity tends to run in families; however, the environment, in the form of what we eat and drink, also plays a significant role in the expression of our genes. Our lifestyle can change our genetic expression! I'll be reviewing epigenetics, how we turn bad genes off and good genes on, in the next chapter.

If sugar is killing us, why do we eat it? The University of Michigan did an interesting study in a preschool. Using mouth swabs, they tested cortisol levels in kids 3-5 years old. They found **stress** affects blood cortisol levels, which increases our appetite and preference for **'comfort' foods** (Lumeng, et al., 2014). Discussing the research (*Colleagues in Care,* March 2012) Lumeng suggests foods with added sugar and high fat actually increase brain opioids causing a soothing effect on the kids and make them feel better. "Three-year old's may not necessarily have a tantrum for a cookie to be manipulative. The cookie may actually make them feel better and reduce their stress." I presented the material on mental health before this chapter as we'll never control our diet until we control stress! "Why do we eat sugar?", often because we're stressed and want to feel better!

I agree with Rich Cohen's, August 2013 National Geographic article, we are "Slaves to Sugar." It's estimated the refinement of sugar cane first occurred about 1000 B.C. and was kept secret, only popping up here and there in the world. About 600 A.D., according to Cohen, the Arab armies "carried away the knowledge and love of sugar."

> It was like throwing paint at a fan: first here and there, sugar turning up wherever Allah was worshipped. Wherever they went, the Arabs brought with them sugar, the product and the technology of its production. Sugar we are told, followed the Koran... the Arabs perfected sugar refinement and turned it into an industry (Cohen, 2013).

Cohen reminds us sugar fueled the slave trade and "It seems like every time I study an illness and trace a path to the first cause, I find my way back to sugar." That is so true! You may want to think about this the next time you indulge in sugar: how Islam perfected sugar refinement, how sugar fueled slave trade and sugars direct link to almost all illness's (including metabolic syndrome). Endocrinologist Dr. Robert Lustig of the University of California says, "Excessive sugar isn't just empty calories, it's **toxic**"!

The University of Michigan study revealed concentrated sugars effect on brain opioids, causing a soothing effect, but, other foods can also affect mood. Casein found in milk, and especially concentrated in cheese, influences endogenous endorphins, which makes dairy products so addictive. In fact, I've had several patients tell me they would rather be overweight than give up milk. Another example of how foods can affect mood is cholecystokinin (CCK). CCK is produced in the gastrointestinal tract in response to fatty foods and results in gallbladder contraction. CCK receptors are also concentrated in the brain and, when stimulated by fatty foods, can result in panic attacks: high fat foods can cause anxiety. We saw in the last chapter how this same chemical can affect pain perception. The point is, foods have an effect on our brain and our thinking! Arby's is not "good mood food", but just the opposite, foods high in fat are bad mood foods. Ellen White addressed this issue years before we understood the science. "The brain and nerves are in sympathy with the stomach. Erroneous eating and drinking result in erroneous thinking and acting" (White, 1910/2004, p.316). Amazing, despite little formal education beyond grade school, Ellen went on during her lifetime to write more than 5,000 periodical articles and 40 books. In **1910** she understood how 'Our Thinking Is Affected By Our Eating'. Unhealthy foods affect us, not only physically, but also mentally.

Rethinking Food

I could make numerous dietary suggestions, but rather than constantly fighting with food, we're going to take a different approach and begin by **rethinking food**. People eat for a variety of reasons. We've all experienced how food can alleviate stress, and a full stomach makes us feel **secure**. In the evenings we often eat for **pleasure**. Many people eat at night to promote **sleep**; however, the wisest man who ever lived, said in Ecclesiastes 5:12, "the sleep of the working man is pleasant, whether he eats little or much. But the full stomach of the rich man does not allow him to sleep." Also, much of our eating is just **habit** and habits are hard to break.

It's so important to evaluate what goes through our mind, as we think about food and food choices – to think about our thinking. Many times I'll be driving home for lunch and suddenly, out of nowhere, I remember left over 'tater tots' in the refrigerator. Where did this come from, I have lots of other healthier foods at home? This came from a stressed brain looking for relief, looking to carbohydrates to relieve my stress! The key is to become aware of our thinking: constantly surveying the landscape of your mind, and evaluating thoughts that come up. Thus, the reason I introduced spirituality in the previous chapters. **Surveying the landscape of your mind** is spirituality and the ability to evaluate your thinking is improved with spiritual disciplines.

Toward the end of a long day we begin to look forward to a big meal; although nothing wrong with this, we need to make sure we're not putting our 'hope' in food. Putting our hope in food, as a stress reliever, is **misplaced hope**! An extremely important life principle is found in Jeremiah 17:5, "**cursed are those who take refuge in the flesh**" (Paraphrased).[10] What's the curse for those who take refuge in, or look forward to, alcohol every night? The curse is often obesity and sometimes alcoholism. What's the curse for those who look forward to drugs every night? Addiction. What is the curse of those who look forward to tobacco? Emphysema and lung cancer. There's nothing wrong with looking forward to a vacation, but, some, by taking refuge in them, have suffered credit card debt and poverty. What's the curse for those who look forward to food? You guessed it, obesity. There's nothing wrong or sinful with looking forward to supper when you're hungry; the point is, we need to look to God for refuge and strength and not to food!

We need to rethink food and what food means to us. The famous chief Emeril Lagasse is famous for saying "**Kick it up a notch**"! He can take an ordinary meal and "kick it up a notch", by adding seasonings or other ingredients, until he's turned ordinary food into the extraordinary. Although nothing necessarily wrong with that, but, is this always necessary? We make food taste so good we simply can't walk away from it! We need to rethink food preparation! Ellen White talks about "Simplicity in diet" avoiding "rich and unhealthful food preparations." C.S. Lewis (1942, p.87) spoke of the "**gluttony of Delicacy**" which is distinct from the "gluttony of excess." We all understand the concept of being gluttonous and eating too much. Lewis is suggesting we can be gluttonous in always expecting delicacies. There really is something to be said about eating fruits and vegetables, as grown, in the way they were designed to be eaten – in their natural "normal and

---

[10] Jeremiah 17:5 NIV - This is what the Lord says: "Cursed is the one who trusts in man, who depends on flesh for his strength and whose heart turns away from the Lord.

humble" state.

We also need to avoid **dietary lies**, food fallacies we've learned. For instance, when the topic of weight loss is introduced, most people immediately respond by discussing exercise. Exercise is extremely important for your overall health, but, is not the answer to weight loss. If we don't focus on the real problem, the number and type of calories we eat, we'll never solve it.

We're told to avoid going too long without food, as this will decrease our metabolism and increase absorption of food the next time we eat, making weight loss more difficult. However, I've never seen any controlled, repeated studies, suggesting this type of extreme change in metabolism after just 10-12 hours of fasting. Another common fallacy is belief that a vegetarian diet will not provide adequate protein and calcium.

Don't be deceived! Look at labels and understand what you're putting into your body. We wouldn't dare stay in a smoke or chemical filled room, breathing toxins; yet, many people eat toxins with little concern. Understand a very sound underlying principle: if man has done anything to food it's usually unhealthy. Finally, I would like to give you a couple motivational thoughts that helped me on my weight loss journey. First, the old English saying, "enough is as good as a feast" Also remember! **"Nothing tastes as good as being thin feels"** (Elizabeth Berg)!

In the 1st century God, in the form of a man, walked the earth and miraculously healed people. Healing still occurs, but, I don't see those kinds of miracles routinely. Today, God has given us knowledge to prevent disease and 'laws of health'. There are laws of health just as sure as the law of gravity!

> Many have expected that God would keep them from sickness merely because they have asked Him to do so…. God will not work a miracle to keep those from sickness who have no care for themselves, but are continually violating the **laws of health**, and make

no effort to prevent disease. . ... God will not work in a miraculous manner to pre-serve the health of persons who are taking a sure course to make themselves sick, by their careless inattention to the laws of health (White, 1914/2004, p312).

Let's review some evidence based, laws of nature, concerning diet and exercise; then, look at proven methods to initiate and maintain a healthy lifestyle.

UPGRADING YOUR LIFESTYLE

What are you "upgrading" in your life at this time? We should always be in a process of continual self-improvement, constantly upgrading our lifestyle, Specifically, we're going to talk about ways of upgrading our diet, and then, in the next section, gradually upgrading activity level. We shouldn't be afraid of growing slow, rather, we need to be afraid of standing still.

Diet Upgrades

Most Americans ingest the **western diet**: high in red meat, sugary desserts, fatty foods, processed meats, refined grains, and dairy products. Most doctors advise patients to upgrade and place us on the **prudent diet**: higher levels of fruits and vegetables, whole grain foods, and more poultry and fish than red meat. Cardiologists try to upgrade this further into the **mediterranean diet** by adding beans and nuts and moderate to high consumption of fish. A **pescetarian die**t upgrades even further, getting closer to a vegetarian diet, which avoids all meat and animal flesh, however, the pescetarian diet allows some seafood. An **ovo-lactarian vegetarian** will not eat any animal flesh or seafood but allows some diary and egg products. Finally, we move up to the **vegan diet**: essentially just fruits, vegetables, nuts, grains, and legumes.

Let's see what the literature has to say about some of these diets.

The PREDIMED trial (Estruch, et al., 2013) broke 7447 people into 3 diets. The 1st two were different types of Mediterranean Diets and the third, a control group, received counseling on a low-fat diet. The two Mediterranean diets, compared with the control low fat group, had a "substantial reduction in the risk of major cardiovascular events." In particular, they were looking at heart attacks, stroke, or deaths from cardiovascular causes. Remember, the classic Mediterranean diet is characterized by a high intake of fruits, vegetables, olive oil, nuts, moderate intake of fish and poultry, but, low intake of red and processed meats, dairy products, and sweets.

Let's take the Mediterranean diet and **upgrade** it to see the effects of the vegetarian diet. The EPIC–Oxford cohort study (Crowe, et al., 2013) looked at 44,561 people. Vegetarians achieve 32% lower risk of ischemic heart disease (blockages of heart arteries). Vegetarians have a 32% lower risk of heart attacks, stents, and bypass surgeries. The EPIC–Oxford cohort study showed a reduction in cardiovascular disease, but, this next study shows a reduced risk of dying with the vegetarian diet, and monitors not just 44,000 people but over 70,000 people.

The **Adventist Health Study – 2** has been going on since 2002 with over 73,000 participants. Out of the project came the *Vegetarian dietary patterns and mortality in Adventist Health Study 2* (Orlich, et al., 2013), which categorized participants into non-vegetarian and 4 different types of vegetarian diets. They were followed for over 5 years during which 2570 deaths occurred. They showed "Vegetarian diets are associated with lower all-cause mortality and with some reductions in cause-specific mortality." Looking at all its other positive qualities, few could doubt the vegetarian diet is the perfect human diet; however, that doesn't mean you need to make a religion out of being vegan, but, **if you don't know where you should be you'll never get there**. We should, at least, be heading in the right direction – constantly upgrading to a plant based diet.

One of the biggest concerns patients raise when discussing a vegan or vegetarian diet is the risk of nutritional deficiency. If you're eating a variety of fruits, vegetables, nuts, and legumes you're not going to be malnourished. However, those strict vegans, who are concerned about preventing nutritional deficiencies should supplement a vitamin B complex, eat beans or tofu, and sprinkle some flaxseed on their food a few times a week.

EXERCISE

"And if being so educated they follow on the same track in their physical training, they will, if they choose, succeed in never needing a doctor except in real necessity" Plato

A fundamental difference between life and non-life (or death) is movement; movement of the organism itself and movement of body fluids. You're never more alive than when you're exercising: the heart is beating harder, moving vital blood and body fluids to tissues which need it. Exercise is vital to life! If you are not exercising you're in a process of slow decay and death, you're dying! In this section, we're going to discuss why exercise is so important, what an appropriate exercise program looks like, and finally, discuss ways of achieving success in diet and exercise by increasing self-control.

We saw how exercise reduces chronic pain and works as well as medications for treatment of depression; in addition, activity was shown to preserve brain volume in older adults! The Cardiovascular Health Study followed 1250 people (all over age 65) for 10 years to determine the risks for developing heart disease and stroke. They were followed very close with yearly measurements of traditional risk factors, such as blood pressure and cholesterol, but also, yearly echocardiograms, carotid ultrasounds, and even brain MRI's. Over 1000 research papers came from this study including one published in the Journal Neuroscience (Braskie et al., 2014). Researchers looked at these brain MRI scans and discovered physical activity preserves brain volume. Actually, their research confirmed several other studies showing "Higher levels of physical activity have been associated with a lower risk of developing Alzheimer's Disease." They showed physical activity also promotes human brain regeneration, including the hippocampus (part of the brain important for memory) and the prefrontal cortex (that part of the brain we determined is so important in developing a healthy lifestyle).

Braskie et al., also pointed out physical activity improves sleep and cardiovascular fitness, resulting in decreased risk of Alzheimer's Disease and brain shrinking. Likewise, confirming lack of physical activity results in obesity, increased body & brain inflammation, and stress, which increases the risk of Alzheimer's Disease and brain shrinkage. Finally, they brought out an interesting and complex relationship between physical activity and stress. Acute physical activity increases cortisol levels, but over time, "decreases the body's (overall) reactivity to stress." We often believe too much stress is dangerous to our health, but, when stress comes three days a week, during strenuous exercise, it turns down the harmful effects of day-to-day stress!

One of the lead researchers, Dr. Cyrus Raji interviewed in *Family Practice News* (2012), suggested "improving lifestyle could reduce the risk for Alzheimer's disease by 50%." He pointed out, "In the United States, the **lack** of physical activity is the No. 1 most powerful lifestyle factor, contributing to 21% of the cases of Alzheimer's disease" and "worldwide, it is the third most powerful risk factor after low educational attainment and smoking." We need to exercise!

UPGRADING YOUR LIFESTYLE

Exercise is extremely important to reduce dependency on the healthcare system. Once again, we're going to look at "upgrading your life."[11] We'll begin with the importance of just getting up and walking, then discuss the benefits of a gradual increasing exercise program. So how far and how fast do we need to go?

Let's begin by discovering how **far** you need to walk to prevent dying! Researchers recorded the distance walked by 707 men and followed for 12 years. The statically significant conclusion was walking over 2 miles a day cuts your death rate in half! "After 12 years of follow-up, 43.1 percent of the men who walked less than one mile per day had died, as compared with 21.5 percent of the men who walked more than two miles per day" (Hakim, et al., 1998). Interestingly, the research showed "Cancer was the most common cause of death; **13.4 percent** of the men who walked less than one mile per day died of cancer, as compared with just **5.3 percent** of those who walked more than two miles per day."

Now, we know how far to walk, but, how **fast** do you need to walk to stay ahead of the Grim Reaper? Researchers followed 1700 men, aged 70 and over: during the study period "no men walking at speeds of 3 miles per hour or above were caught by Death" (Stanaway, et al., 2011). The researchers suggest, "This supports the hypothesis that faster speeds are protective against mortality because fast walkers can maintain a safe distance from the Grim Reaper." So, to avoid death we need to walk at least 2 miles a day and maintain walking speeds over 3 miles an hour.

Let's see how things change when we step-up the pace a bit. Studenski et al., 2011, also proved "gait speed was associated with survival in older adults"; however, they showed the intensity of exercise and overall survival are 'dose related'. At every age, the faster the walking "dose" the longer the individual lives! We're

---

[11] I would like to acknowledge the exercise research bibliography presented by Barry A. Franklin PhD (Congdon lecture 2014)

interested in the effects of **upgrading our lifestyle,** as we don't want to just survive. Let's look at the effects of "walking compared to vigorous exercise for the prevention of cardiovascular disease" (heart attack and strokes).

Manson et al., 2002, showed the more we upgrade the exercise program, the more "vigorous" the exercise program becomes, the lower our risk of cardiovascular disease. Their study looked at over 73,000 people between the ages of 50 to 79 and showed "An increasing physical-activity score had a strong, graded, inverse association with the risk of both coronary events and total cardiovascular events." They also showed a corresponding improvement in insulin sensitivity as the level of exercise intensity increased; which, as we discovered, is so important in metabolic syndrome. Finally, they confirmed "physical activity of any intensity has been linked to improvement in emotional well-being."

A study by the American Heart Association (Kokkinos et al., 2008) showed a proportionate lower risk for **all causes** of death as you increase your activity level. Interestingly, they showed the influence of exercise was more important than other risk factors such as high blood pressure, diabetes, cholesterol, and smoking.

> Our findings support a strong inverse and graded reduction in mortality risk with increased exercise capacity. In accordance with recent reports, we found that *exercise capacity was a more powerful predictor of risk for all-cause mortality than established risk factors* among both blacks and whites after adjustment for cardiac medications and traditional CVD risk factors.

If indeed, exercise is more important in preventing death than hypertension, diabetes, and cholesterol, one would ask why this is not the primary agenda in our healthcare system. At least part of the answer is financial. Drug companies and the healthcare systems don't make money if you prevent disease by exercising and eating right – **they** survive the healthcare crisis only if **you** take medications and struggle to survive!

Understanding just how important exercise is, let's look at the four components of an exercise program: **cardiovascular** work-out, **stretching, strength** training and, especially for older people, **balance** training.

Cardiovascular

Other than walking or jogging outside, I would suggest using a treadmill for your cardiovascular work-out. As a 'rule of thumb', it's been recommended we get our heart rate over 120, for 20 minutes, at least three days a week. Treadmills provide feedback which motivates us to upgrade our activity. Treadmills don't pound on your joints like road running, and it's easier to adjust environmental temperature when you're inside. Some people like the elliptical machine or exercise bike, however, **treadmills are much more physiologic**. I suggest walking and running, as our legs were created, and balanced, for these activities. Nothing particularly wrong with other types of work-outs, if you get your heart rate up; however, I worry about disturbing the correct balance of muscles across leg joints, perhaps leading to arthritis. Also, as we get to extremes of age, we often just want to maintain postural muscles (the ability to stand-up and walk). To maintain our ability to walk, we need to exercise walking and running muscles.

Starting an exercise program is more about time management than anything else. At the beginning of each week, look at your schedule and commit 30 minutes, three days a week to exercise. If your schedule only provides for a 4am work-out, then, so be it! At the beginning of your **lifetime** exercise journey, it's not so much what you do, just do something for 30 minutes, three times a week. If all you can do is walk, then just walk for 30 minutes. Exercise intensity will naturally increase as you go along. Keep a journal, writing down how far, how fast, and how long you've walked. Slowly, even if it's just for 20 seconds, increase the pace to a brisk walk or even a slow jog. As time goes on, you'll progress to jogging 30 minutes, 3 times a week, and your life will change! Think of the awesome gift you could give yourself, even if it took 5 years to develop. Maintain a **lifetime** exercise perspective; you need be on "the 50-year plan"! Therefore, it's not so much what you do each day, just commit those three days a week, for the rest of your life! You'll need to walk 60 minutes **every day**, if it's impossible, not just improbable, for you to jog. Most people, however, don't have 60 free minutes; so, you'll need to slowly build up your work-out intensity.

Jogging gets easier, but never gets easy. There's a certain amount of suffering inherent in life; you can divide it up in small aliquots, on the treadmill, 3 times a week, or get it all at once, in intensive care units during the end stages of your life. I can promise, exercise will change your life! Stress melts away and for many people it's the cure for depression! You'll feel so much better and your self-esteem sky-rockets! You'll sleep better and have more energy during the day. Your natural pain killers (endorphins) are built up, so you experience less overall pain. However, exercise, especially jogging, is hard work. So, the other thing I can promise, during your work-out, you'll sometimes feel like you're dying! This feeling is scary, so we lie to ourselves, believing this activity may somehow be harming us. Therefore, you need to "**run like you're not afraid of dying but be prepared in case you do**"!

A well-meaning orthopedic surgeon, when asked if jogging causes arthritis, suggested our knees are like car tires which can wear out. He's wrong! Our joints are nothing like car tires. Joints are living tissue with the ability for self-repair, if conditions are right. It's not runners I see getting joint replacements, but more often, it's over weight individuals who didn't exercise! In fact, research has shown a rigorous 12-week exercise program in patients with severe hip arthritis reduced the number of artificial hip replacements (Svege, et al., 2013). Leading researcher, Linda Fernandes PhD, says the take home message is "Don't be afraid of your pain. It won't damage your cartilage" (Otto, 2011).

Stretching is the "fountain of youth"

As you begin your exercise program, there will be occasions when your back will hurt, your knees will hurt, your hips will hurt, your ankles will hurt: the list goes on and on. Whatever hurts, stretch it! Stretch for 10-15 minutes before and sometimes after each run. During well-child exams, I always ask the kids to bend down and touch their toes. The kids often stay in this bent posture and the parents will say "ok you can stand up now." They stay bent over because it feels good! Stretching releases endorphins, natural "feel good" chemicals, into your body.

I've seen numerous elderly patients, suffering from neck arthritis, unable to turn their head more than 20 degrees. At what point did the neck "suddenly" become unable to turn? A daily neck stretching program will help maintain range of motion, even across very tiny neck joints, reducing and preventing the pain of arthritis. I suggest a very simple routine everyone can do. Each morning, sit at your bedside, and stretch your neck, shoulders, and low back. Also, three times a week, during your exercise program, lie down and stretch your legs.

The balance across a joint is extremely important. Not only should muscles stay balanced by doing physiologic exercises, such as walking and running, also, ligaments and tendons across joints should remain balanced and flexible. For instance, if the hamstrings (behind the knee) tighten up, it will bend the knee, ever so slightly, causing weight loads to shift toward the back of the knee, altering forces across the joint. Think of an older person who walks stooped over, with knees slightly bent and leaning forward at the hips. Tissues behind the knee, and in front of the hip, have tightened down into a contracture. Now they walk in this stooped posture, which can wear down joints, throw off balance and increase the risk of falling.

It's very important to properly strengthen and stretch joints to maintain balance!

Exercise physiologists suggest many people in developed countries are unable to squat. Squatting to have a bowel movement, for example, is as natural as life itself; however, this position is lost in "developing" countries with the use of toilets. Squatting stretches the quadricep muscles and strengthens the ankles, helping to prevent arthritis. It's very interesting how the 'kneeling down', posture of prayer, has also been lost in many cultures. This position properly stretches, not only our knees and back, but also, our spirits. I wonder how many chronic back, hip, and knee problems would be prevented, and even cured, by kneeling daily before the Lord?

Strength Training

We've discussed the importance of cardiovascular conditioning and stretching, however, strength training (muscle building) cannot be neglected. I've referred to insulin receptors (the locks which insulin keys fit into) and how important it is to keep those locks functioning well. Strength training builds new insulin receptors on muscle, but, those receptors down regulate (melt away) after just 4 days of inactivity. Therefore, strength training should occur at least twice a week. Torn shoulder muscles (rotator cuff), are a major problem as we age. Stretching and properly strengthening shoulder muscles will help prevent rotator cuff tears. However, I would avoid repetitious overhead ("shoulder-press") movements, which cause rotator cuff problems! Rather, I would suggest the "fly" and "chest press" for upper body strengthening. Use the upper body for strength training and reserve the legs only for your walking/running cardiovascular work-out.

Balance Training

Especially as we age, we need to introduce balance training into our work-out routine. Maintaining posture and balance is truly amazing, as many body systems function together for equilibrium;

including the inner ear, vision, and stretch receptors in muscles and tendons; all under the control of a part of the brain called the cerebellum. These balance mechanisms, like other aging organ systems, can fail us resulting in balance problems, chronic dizziness and instability which leads to falling. Balance training becomes very important as we age! The physical act of Ti Chi is an excellent way to develop and maintain balance. I've discussed balance across weight bearing joints and a complete exercise program which balances us physiologically; however, we need balance in body, mind, and spirit. Ellen White (1884/2004, p311) wrote about balance and harmony,

> The harmonious, healthy action of all the powers of body and mind results in happiness; the more elevated and **refined** the powers, the more pure and unalloyed the happiness. An aimless life is a living death. The mind should dwell upon themes relating to our eternal interests. This will be conducive to health of body and mind.

SELF CONTROL: THE ULTIMATE BALANCING ACT

Our diet and work-out schedule requires harmony and balance of body, mind, and spirit; however, perseverance requires self-control. Self-control, as suggested in Miller and Rollnick's concept of *Motivational Interviewing*, often plays out as a balance between "indulgence and restraint." In doing a systematic review of motivational interviewing Rubak et al., (2005), states "Ambivalence takes the form of a conflict between two courses of action (i.e. indulgence and restraint), each has perceived benefits and costs associated with it." They're suggesting our lack of self-control comes from ambivalence. However, as you will see below, God can interact with us individually, guiding us through the process of eliciting, clarifying, and resolving ambivalence to change.

Ellen White (2004, p295) wrote, "One of the most deplorable effects of the original apostasy", referring to the fall in the Garden of Eden, "was that people lost the power of **self-control**. Only as this power is regained can there be real progress." All day long people present to my office suffering, in misery and in despair: relationship problems, depression, pain, patients who've suffered strokes, heart attacks and endured bypass surgeries. As a physician, at least 80% of the conditions I treat on a daily basis, all come down to self-control!

"If I had a **pill for self-control**," I once suggested, "I'd be the richest man who ever lived." However, reality presented itself when I meet Lisa. Suffering with tobacco and alcohol abuse, she came to my office looking for addictions to Vicodin and Xanax. I held out my hand, pretending to have a pill to increase self-control. I told Lisa if she took this pill she would never want to smoke or drink alcohol again. She made the sign of a cross with her fingers, as if pushing away a vampire, saying "get it away." I quickly realized there would never be a pill for self-control.

Like love, joy, and peace, I've learned self-control (including control of lifestyle, diet, and exercise) is the 'fruit' of a developing spiritual life. Recall, Viktor Frankl wrote, "The spiritual dimension cannot be ignored, for it is what makes us human." What makes us human is our ability for higher thinking, which is spirituality. As we develop spiritually, we manifest uniquely human characteristics, such as love and joy, peace and patience, kindness, gentleness, and goodness. We learn about these *Fruits of the Spirit*, fruits of a developing spiritual life, in the book of Galatians, chapter 5. These fruits are characteristics which make us uniquely human. Galatians 5 tells us another unique human attribute is **self-control**! Self-control, the fruit of a developing spiritual, thinking existence, allows us to take-control of diet and exercise, and overcoming harmful habits. The fruits of peace and patience reduces stress, which drains us of energy required to effectively diet and exercise.

What's prevented you from developing the lifestyle you want? Exercise is difficult. It's easier to take a pill for cholesterol and sugar than diet. It's much harder, and takes two hands, to push away the dinner plate away, and takes two feet, to begin walking or jogging. **However, being empowered by Kingdom of God spirituality will allow you to manifest the fruit of self-control to accomplish your goals.**

MOVING FROM PRINCIPLE TO PRAXIS
"You will show me the **path of life**" Psalm 16:11

The stage is set. We've come to the central and most critical part of the entire book. It's time to *Heal the Heart from the Inside Out!* We've seen the importance of understanding our complete nature (improved health by understanding self). We've seen the importance of clarifying our belief systems, before lasting behavioral changes occur (beliefs bubble out into behavior). I've shown how spirituality clarifies true mental health, and gets us above the plane of pain. Now, we're prepared to embrace a healthy lifestyle, as we journey into the next chapter of the book, and our lives, *Graceful Aging*.

To assist in our transformational journey, we've employed the concepts of transformational learning. We've seen how spirituality builds the scaffolding needed for self-reflection and perspective transformation. Likewise, understanding our complete nature (body, mind, and spirit), we're free to use, not only rational **insights, judgments, and decisions**; but **symbols, images, and feelings** which <u>motivate</u> us to change.

Spirituality is a critical element in transformation! Indeed, before we can make lasting changes we must look at our belief systems and analyze our values. Ellen White (2004, p302) tells us "A person whose mind is quiet and satisfied in God is in the **pathway** to health." The battle for weight control and motivation to exercise, is not just a battle for self-control but a battle to stay quiet and satisfied in God! By dwelling on spiritual matters your life becomes invigorated and directed. Psalm 16: 8 & 11 are key verses in disease prevention: "Because I have set the LORD continually before me; I will not be shaken…. He will make known to me the **path of life**" (paraphrased). By concentrating on spiritual issues (setting the LORD always before you), you will be guided into the right way of living (path of life), a path unique to you and your current situation.

The "path of life" is unique to everyone. A relationship with God will help clarify your personal strengths and weaknesses as you discover your ability to change. Again, we see commonalities between the biblical "**path of life**" and the concept of motivational interviewing. Rubak points out, "Readiness to change is not a client trait, but a fluctuating product of interpersonal interaction." Change is the product of an 'interpersonal interaction' with God though the person of Jesus the Christ. A proper relationship with God is one which respects the individuals "intrinsic values and goals to stimulate behavior change." It's difficult to arouse and maintain motivation to change from within ourselves, but develops naturally within this kind of relationship!

The "path of life" is unique to everyone; we're guided along that path, only as our spirit joins with Gods Holy Spirit. As the Holy Spirit came upon the disciples in the 2nd chapter of Acts, Peter shouts "You have revealed the **paths of life** to me." The Greek word for "paths" is "hodos," which means a way (manner) of feeling, thinking and deciding. Hodos, the path of life, the way of life, is a lifestyle. True health is not something you can strive to achieve, it must come naturally, it must be who you are. Christians are health, they are life! Lifestyle comes from within, it comes from who you are. As you will see in the next chapter, it even changes who you are genetically!

The apostle Paul's revealed the answer to his problem with self-control in Roman's 8, "For those who are according to the flesh set their **minds** on the flesh but those who are according to the **spirit** the things of the spirit. For the mind set on the flesh is **death** but the mind set on the spirit is **life** and peace..." He goes on to write, "**If by the Spirit** you are putting to death the deeds of your body you will live." Are you thinking only about things around you, the things you can see, or using your brain, your mind, your spirit, to think about realities unseen?

I've shown how the metacognitive (thinking about your thinking) view of spirituality gets us out of the mental illness **trap**, the chronic pain **trap** and now out of the physical **trap** called metabolic syndrome. Like a maze, it's easier to get out if you can get to higher ground and see the dead-ends. To get out of these traps we need to develop the **ability** for higher level thinking – to think about our thinking. Spirituality increases our ability for self-reflection; to look back upon ourselves and our experiences. You've now arrived at a precipice, a cliff, a point where you can look at your life, evaluate your lifestyle, see the dead-ends, and make the course adjustments needed. Spirituality gives us the ability to **survey the landscape of our mind** and make the vital changes needed.

CHAPTER 6

GRACEFUL AGING

Cling to Him, for He is your **life** and the **length** of your days
(Deuteronomy 30:20)

When we're young, aging seems to occur so slowly, it's easy to neglect the reality of it. Work, family, and other responsibilities, are so pressing we sometimes put off healthy lifestyles. In fact, many destroy their lives, just trying to "make end meets." Spirituality helps us work through the demands of life and still maintain our health. The wisest man who ever lived said, "**Remember your Creator in the days of your youth**, before the days of trouble come and the years approach when you will say, 'I find no pleasure in them'" Ecclesiastes 12:1. We must take time to prepare for the aging process. Indeed, we need to take time to remember our Creator in the days of our youth, as only through God's "grace" can we meet all the requirements of today and still prepare for tomorrow. Thus, the reason I've entitled this chapter "graceful" aging rather than "healthy" aging.

We've looked at disease prevention. However, none of us are getting out of here alive, so, unless the LORD returns, or we die suddenly, we'll all struggle with the eventual decay of our physical life. However, when the dean of my medical school, presented the first lecture, he suggested the goal of medicine is to "square off the curve" of this health decay. He was referring to the slow downward curve our health can take, over years, leading to disease and disability. Dean Myron Magen suggested our goal, as physicians, is to keep people healthy until just before death; thus, **"squaring off the curve."** My goal in this chapter is to shorten this process of health decay from years to just days, or even hours, before death!

Poor lifestyle choices result in the slow decay of our body into debility. Also, a **fear of death and dying** can prolong the process, leading to a "slow decay." To reduce this fear, we'll look at the natural process of death and dying and review the importance of advance directives. We'll then go on to look at theories of aging and anti-aging techniques.

DEATH AND DYING

I've heard people say, "I hope I die in my sleep." Yet, I've never seen anyone die who was not "in their asleep." Unless we die suddenly from a traumatic accident or acute medical problem, we'll all die "in our sleep." Whether we succumb to heart disease, cancer, stroke, pneumonia, or some other disease, often, the immediate cause of death centers around the effects of dehydration (regardless of the cause, we eventually become too weak to eat and drink). It's important to understand, however, we don't die of thirst or hunger. It's interesting, how our sense of thirst decreases as we age. Studies depriving both younger and older people of water have shown the elderly tolerate dehydration much better than younger people. That's one reason older people need to monitor their fluid intake and make sure to purposely drink enough and not wait on thirst: a principle very important for your overall health.

To demystify and reduce fear, let's look at the experience of dying. Humans can live a month or more without food, but only a week or two without water. Although we don't 'starve to death' or 'die of thirst' most of us will, ultimately, succumb to the effects of dehydration. Several biological events come together in the natural dying process. Dehydration reduces kidney function which increases sodium and potassium in the blood. The sodium imbalance acts as a **natural anesthetic**, making the person sleepy, which further reduces their fluid intake. A progressive cycle of dehydration, sodium increases, and lethargy occurs, leading to a state of unconsciousness. All the while, blood potassium levels go higher and higher, eventually stopping the heart, and the person dies, "in their sleep", naturally and painlessly. In my experience, this final event of dying "in our sleep" occurs over a 2-3-day period. Interestingly, Jewish people call such a dying individual a "goses."

Per Jewish tradition, "a goses is a patient who would be described by people working in end- of-life care today as 'actively dying.' This state has been defined in Jewish texts as existing during the last 3 or so days of a person's life" (Kinzbrunner, 2002). In describing this respectful dying process, Lois Stanely from Temple Beth El suggests, "We do everything to save life- *pikuch nefesh*, but once the boundary has been crossed into goses, we must not unnaturally prolong the dying. One must die with comfort with dignity and sanctity" (Congdon Lecture Series).

It's helps to know the experience of dying, the experience of a goses, is God directed! Also, there's nothing morally wrong with just **saying no**! If you don't want a treatment, especially one which is just going to prolong the inevitable, just say no. In many situations, by saying no, you're opening the door for the medical system to provide comfort! But, is it legal to die?

IS IT LEGAL TO DIE?

This may sound like a silly question, but many people are kept alive with feeding tubes and other unnatural medical interventions against their will. For them, it's not legal to die! Some people, without advance directives, become a "ward of the court" or have a court appointed guardian. Under most circumstances, the court will not "pull the plug." The government cannot terminate life or with-hold treatment to one of its citizens. In these, and other unique circumstances, it's not legal to die.

I hate to see a medical "system" prolong a person in a "vegetative-like" state or in a situation the individual finds unacceptable. Feeding tubes, for example, are "easy" to put in but difficult to remove. After all, who wants to remove a feeding tube, depriving someone of their only source of water and nutrition? It's one thing to allow nature to take its course, allowing the person to die a natural death, but another thing entirely to remove a tube the person's life is now dependent on.

I had an opportunity to care for an entire nursing home, for over a decade, and learned many valuable lessons on aging, death & dying, and the importance of advance directives. At the beginning of my nursing home career, an 80-year-old patient was admitted after a stroke. She was losing weight, and yet, refused a feeding tube. I brought the case to my Family Medicine department meeting, concerned about the ethical and possible legal implications. Essentially, I was asking the other physicians if it was ethical and legal to die! The physicians were unanimous. She had the right to refuse treatment and let nature take its course. However, there needs to be advance directives.

For years, the medical community used the phrase "D.N.R." (Do Not Resuscitate). Now, we're starting to use the term "A.N.D." (Allow Natural Death); an important distinction, especially for family members struggling to make difficult end of life decisions. The designation "Do Not Resuscitate" suggests we're deciding to let someone die, whereas, "Allow Natural Death" places this decision in the hands of God. A 'DNR' order suggests we're not doing something (we're not resuscitating), whereas 'AND' removes guilt, suggesting we're letting nature take its course.

The current legal environment allows any adult to refuse treatment, if they can make intelligent and informed decisions. However, toward the end of life, most people depend on a Medical Durable Power of Attorney (MDPOA). MDPOA forms are easily obtained from any hospital or doctor's office, free of charge. The form simply asks the individual's name and the name of two other people who would make decisions for them if necessary. Usually the form requires all parties sign the paper with two witnesses. Studies have shown appropriate advance directives decrease the time required for establishment of comfort care goals and avoids protracted dying (Campbell and Guzman, 2003).

Often these difficult, end of life decisions, come down to worldview. For example, if a person comes to the end of life, believing heaven awaits, and can say with the apostle Paul, "For to me, to live is Christ and to die is gain", they're usually spared the life prolonging, sometimes painful procedures, and allowed to die in peace. However, if this life is all there is, sometimes decisions are made to prolong that life, regardless of the suffering the person must endure.

Too often, as we approach the end of life, one hospital stay and procedure gradually turns into another. Family members (or caregivers) directing decisions start to wonder if they're only prolonging things, and maybe, even causing unnecessary suffering. On the other hand, we feel obligated to save the life of the person we love. The truth is, no matter what we do or don't do, it's hard to feel comfortable when the end of life is near. We need to let God be the God of life and death, and place the person in His caring hands. How do we develop the sense of trust and courage needed during this challenging time?

THE MATURATION OF FEAR vs. TRUST

Most people call them nursing homes, healthcare workers call them extended care facilities, while some residents claimed to be in the 'county poor farm'. Regardless of the name, it's often a place of extremes: extremes of age, poverty, illness, emotions, and sometimes even suffering. Yet, it's surprising to see how desperately many hold onto life.

You would expect someone, who has struggled for decades to live, wouldn't suddenly give-up on life, and yet, this tenacity for living sometimes goes beyond a healthy respect for life. Many elderly people endure unbelievable suffering, just to squeeze out a couple more drops of life, sometimes, due to a fear of death! In the extreme end of life there seems to be two kinds of people: those who grew with each problem, gaining strength and trust, but also, those individuals who never grew, each struggle just adding to their burden and bitterness. Their **fears matured** throughout life into a nightmarish situation!

When reality sets in, the process of death & dying may seem scary. However, much of what happens depends on whether, throughout life, we've matured fear or trust. I certainly don't believe God intends his children to die a slow painful death, when heaven is just around the corner! Yet, many people, unsure of the afterlife, are afraid to die and simply prolong the process, believing this life maybe all there is. How sad! How sad, these same individuals didn't show this tenacity for life, when they were younger, in the form of healthy lifestyles, disease prevention and a search for truth! Unfortunately, at the end, when everything is truly lost and facing eternity, they hold onto life with everything they have, because of a fear of death, a fear of God, whom many choose to ignore their entire life. When everything is said and done, the person pays a terrible price in pain and discomfort, simply to add a few weeks of life. Others, 'believed' in God, but chose to live for themselves: chasing idols of money, status, bigger houses, and better cars, and now they know judgment awaits!

I once cared for a man in his late 80's who developed deep ulcers on both legs, with no hope of recovery. Having multiple chronic conditions, he was unable to walk or care for himself, requiring 24 hour a day attendants. He quit eating, was malnourished, and when given the option, requested a feeding tube. Concerned about the quality of his life, I wanted to make sure he was making an informed decision. Recall, it's easy to start tube feedings, but hard to stop when the person's life is now dependent upon it. After educating him, he understood, and still wanted the feeding tube. I'd never seen anyone struggle so hard for life, in the face of death. I asked him about his thoughts concerning life after death, to which he replied, **"I never really thought about it."**

I encountered another elderly man, in the nursing home, who was miserable despite excellent care. He was very angry and unhappy. I tried to add hope to his life, and simply asked if he ever thought about heaven. Even on his deathbed, this retired farmer, told me he didn't believe in God. "Where do you think you came from," I asked; to which, he replied, "my mom."

Here we see two men, both living 80 plus years. One never really thought about God or heaven, the other, flippantly ignored any abstract reasoning about life itself. Neither man showing any respect for the mysterious nature of life, let alone their own origin! Are you going to be an 80-year-old, who spent more time trying to understand how your car came into being, then you did trying to understand how you came to be? Are you more interested in the stock market then life itself? How embarrassing to live 80 years, and near the end say, "I never really thought about it." What's your best guess?

Enough about death and dying. Death is **not** something to be feared. Most of us will die "in our sleep." **The important thing is to be prepared with advance directives, not only for this life, but also, advance directives for the life to come**!

HEALTHSPAN vs. LIFESPAN

Let's change directions and talk about healthy aging. Our goal is to match our healthspan with our lifespan: to stay healthy, and maintain a high functional capacity, until just before death. Unfortunately, many start the gradual decline into infirmity in their mid-30's, resulting in a process of slow decay into death; experiencing a difference between their health span and lifespan. We develop a certain lifestyle in our 20's, which seems very natural and well tolerated. However, after the age 30 this lifestyle can cause our health span and lifespan to slowly separate.

At what age, do we start to age? A newborn baby's tissues are not oxidizing and decaying. Many believe our tissues start to breakdown about the age 30 or 33. Thankfully, our bodies can recover from a lot of abuse delivered during our teen years and twenties. It becomes much harder, after age 30, to recover from these insults and imbalances imposed on our body.

Increasing lifespan is something most happy and healthy people strive for. However, if your health (your healthspan) reduces too quickly you'll become dependent on others, and dependent on the healthcare system, for the remainder of your lifespan. Again, the important thing is to "square off" the curve, staying healthy until just before death. I'm suggesting staying healthy until just hours before death, or a couple of days, at the longest.

Years ago, people didn't live long enough to notice a drop in their healthspan. Infectious disease caused many to die, at a young age, before chronic conditions like diabetes, heart disease and stroke occurred. Interestingly, our improved lifespan, resulting from a reduction in infectious disease, wasn't due to antibiotics. Our increased lifespan came from immunizations, improved sanitation, and nutrition. Our improved **life**span didn't come from the healthcare system; likewise, our improved **health**span will not come from a pill. Improved **health**span comes from improved nutrition and lifestyle. Of course, this isn't something pharmaceutical companies are going to tell you, and it's often neglected by our busy healthcare system. The process of prolonging our healthspan, to match a longer lifespan, is not about improved healthcare but improved **self-care**!

Still too often, we're convinced pills are the answer. Antiaging has become a big market. Hormone replacement, vitamins, herbs, antioxidants, and dietary supplements have become big business. "The number of testosterone prescriptions written in the U.S. grew nearly tenfold from 2000 to 2011, part of a worldwide boom" (Von Drehle, 2014). Unfortunately, if we rely only on medications, there will always be a gap between our healthspan and lifespan.

THEORIES OF AGING

Throughout this book, I've emphasized the importance of brain and cognitive health, both essential for the metacognitive development of spirit. Therefore, as we review the various theories of aging I'll concentrate specifically on the sustenance of brain health, as even subtle insults can become so profound. Aging is a very complex phenomenon, but research often centers around 4 major factors: excess insulin, elevated blood sugar, uncontrolled free radicals, and epigenetic changes. Let's briefly examine each one.

Excess Insulin

We saw the damaging effects of insulin in the last chapter. To quickly review: weight gain creates elevated insulin levels, resulting in body tissues becoming resistant to insulin. Insulin **resistance** elevates blood pressure and cholesterol, also, because the body becomes resistant to the effects of insulin, blood sugar goes up. These are just a few of the numerous deleterious effects of high insulin levels which, ultimately, results in aging.

Willette et al., (2015), using functional PET scans of the brain, to detect the adverse effects of insulin, point out, "Several studies indicate that peripheral insulin resistance and related conditions, such as metabolic syndrome and diabetes mellitus, are risk factors for cognitive decline and Alzheimer's Disease and are linked with an increased risk for death from dementia."

Elevated Blood Sugar

Glucose (blood sugar) itself is often touted as a mechanism of aging. Suji & Sivakami (2004) even suggest "glucose seems to be central to the phenomenon of aging and age-related diseases." Diabetics are familiar with the glycohemoglobin lab, which tells how well their blood sugar was controlled in the prior 3-month period. Sugar attaches to the oxygen carrying hemoglobin molecule. After measuring the amount of sugar on the hemoglobin protein, which is replaced every 3 months, we discover the average blood sugar. Importantly, sugar also attaches to other proteins, throughout the body, accelerating the aging process.

Sugar can also attach to brain proteins resulting in "Advanced Glycated End products" (AGE's). Brain proteins don't renew every three months, like red blood cells. Therefore, these glycated proteins accumulate in brain tissue. Yaffe et al., (2011) showed, how increased AGE levels are "linked to age-related conditions including inflammation, vascular disease, and chronic kidney disease" but more importantly, advanced glycated end products "accelerated cognitive aging."

In the previous chapter, we looked at various types of diets, without looking at the total number of calories. Now, as we look specifically at anti-aging, we need to introduce the concept of **caloric restriction** (reducing the total number of calories in our diet). Caloric restriction has been called the "Holy Grail" of anti-aging. Barry Sears (1999) writes, "In fact, in every animal species ever tested, restricting calorie intake has always produced a longer and a more functional life with less chronic disease." Sears goes on to suggest, "there is only one consensus in the world of anti-aging: the only proven way to reverse aging is to restrict calories."

We certainly cannot turn back the hands of time. There's no wonder drug to slow aging. However, caloric restriction, eating less without malnutrition, has been proven to slow the aging process. Being under nourished is different from being malnourished. Food intake, beyond what is essential, stokes the fire which burns and ages your body. High blood sugar accelerates aging. Suji & Sivakami (2004) suggest "caloric restriction, which is known to prolong life span, appears to act by bringing about mild hypoglycemia and increased insulin sensitivity."

Uncontrolled Free Radicals

Let's move on and look at the free radical/oxidative stress theory of aging. We hear a lot about **antioxidants** which clear the body of damaging oxygen free radicals. Oxygen free radicals come from numerous things, such as pollution, smoking, and even sunlight. More importantly, for our purposes, oxygen free radicals come from the foods we eat. Free radicals normally develop from the breakdown of food into energy. Thankfully, we have natural antioxidant systems to handle this oxidative stress. However, our free radical savaging systems are overwhelmed when we eat too much, or eat too much of the wrong kind of foods. Also, as we age, our bodies normal antioxidant systems may become less effective. Bokov et al., (2004) showed **caloric restriction** "reduces the age-related increase in oxidative damage to biomolecules." Kasapis and Thompson (2005) suggest, "there is evidence that long-term **physical activity** increases antioxidant defenses through the up-regulation of antioxidant enzymes."

Caloric restriction has a positive effect on the body; but again, let's specifically look at the effects of caloric restriction on the brain. Consider the concept of **mental energy**. **Neuroenergetics** (brain energy) is important as we look at cognitive and memory loss, often associated with aging. Brain energy comes from microscopic intracellular "power plants" we call mitochondria. The brain has the highest energy demands of any organ based on size, so it's very important that brain cell mitochondria stay functional.

> Mitochondrial function declines with age in the brain and has been proposed to be a major factor in the loss of brain function with aging.... As a result, preserving brain mitochondrial integrity and metabolism with age could be critical for maintaining healthy brain function (Lin et al., 2014)

They also suggest caloric restriction slows the age-related decline of brain mitochondrial function. "These results provide a rationale for caloric restriction-induced sustenance of brain health with extended lifespan." There's no doubt restricting the number of calories you take in, helps to slow the aging process, both physically and cognitively. However, one of the newest and most important aging and anti-aging theories is epigenetics!

Epigenetics

Every cell in the body contains the exact same chromosomes (our inheritance); so, why do some cells become a heart cell and some a brain cell? Although they all contain the same chromosomal material, only certain types of genetic information is turned on in the various cells. Therefore, some cells become part of the heart and some part of the brain. Human cells have 23 pairs of chromosomes. When unraveled, a chromosome simply contains a single strand of DNA, about 3 meters long, which codes for our genetic make-up; for instance, the color of our eyes. DNA is carefully spun around spools of proteins called histones, much like spools of thread. Scattered throughout these 23 pairs of chromosomes are about 25,000 "genes" we inherent from both parents which determine some of our unique personal characteristics.

For years, scientists thought all genes were frozen and unchangeable. However, through the study of epigenetics, we've learned to influence how **active** certain genes are. Scientists now understand these histone spools also act as switches, capable of turning some genes on and off. There are "epigenetic factors" which influence the histones tails, opening or closing certain genes; promoting or reducing cancer, autoimmune conditions (like lupus and rheumatoid arthritis), even effecting mental illness and diabetes. In fact, it's been estimated only 50% of what we are, is controlled solely by our inheritance, the other 50% by epigenetics – which we can influence by our lifestyle.

As an example of the power of epigenetics, researchers looked at an isolated area in Sweden where starvation and feasting, were dependent on crop growth. Bygren et al., (2001), showed the offspring of people born during years of gluttony lived shorter lives. Epigenetics, however, isn't just about influencing our offspring, as some genes are turned on and off even during our lives and influence the aging process.

ANTI-AGING

Geroprotectors are interventions used to slow aging and extend healthspan and lifespan. We're going to review how lifestyle geroprotectors, such as exercise, diet, maintenance of circadian rhythms, and mental health, are capable of influencing epigenetics and aging. **I will ultimately go on to show how the type of thinking you have can influence aging even at this genetic level.**

First, let's look at the effects of *exercise* on gene expression and aging. We all understand how lack of activity results in weakness; therefore, because we're weak, we're less active and grow even weaker (a vicious cycle develops). However, there's more to the story. When we don't exercise, our body shifts from a very efficient way of burning fuel to a very inefficient way. This new, inefficient, way of burning fuel, causes more free radical production which accelerates aging. The problem grows worse! Gregory Brewer, in the journal Experimental Gerontology (2010) suggests, **when we enter** a sedentary lifestyle, we make epigenetic changes resulting in insulin resistance, with all the associated problems, such as high blood pressure and cholesterol. In short, these "epigenetic changes" lead to accelerated aging. **The way out** of this cycle is exercise and diet!

Orozco & Sassone (2014), showed how *caloric restriction* results in epigenetic changes, ultimately, leading to healthy aging. Interestingly, they also suggested a correlation between epigenetics and circadian rhythms! Strategies focused at controlling circadian rhythm, for example, regular sleep schedules and low caloric scheduled meals, might beneficially influence the negative effects of aging.

A regular lifestyle, i.e. scheduled sleep cycles, meals, and exercise, all have a powerful influence on aging (Cornelissen and Otsuka, 2016). We've all experienced the power of circadian rhythms, as we tend to awake at the same time every day. Like many things which go wrong as we age, our circadian rhythms also decline. Brown et al., (2011), showed therapies aimed at sustaining circadian function increased quality of life in the elderly.

There's a rhythm to life, a certain harmony and balance to youthfulness, we seem to lose as we grow older. Body temperature, urine volume, blood pressure and even brain blood flow all have rhythms. Hormones such as cortisol, sex hormones, growth hormone and numerous others are released in waves, in cyclic patterns. In fact, there's been shown to be a cyclic mechanism to antioxidants. The accumulation of all these cycles results in the perfect harmony and balance of life. Unfortunately, "there's erosion in the robustness of the circadian rhythms during aging" (Orozco & Sassone, 2014). Aging is a loss of harmony – **we lose the rhythm of life**. "Disturbances in the circadian clock have been associated to various pathologies including, obesity, type-2 diabetes, eating disorders, sleep disorders, Alzheimer's disease and psychiatric disorders (even) cancer and memory reduction" (Ibid).

Why do so many people die shortly after they retire? They got out of rhythm with themselves. Rhythm is so important in life. It's not just staying in tune to our **personal** circadian cycles; even **life** itself has many cycles. Look at the menstrual cycle, responsible for the propagation of life! What about the effect seasons have on hibernation, nesting, and mating? **Creation** also has cycles. Look at lunar cycles and the massive effect it has over the oceans. How does all this tie into the weekly Sabbath: the ultimate rhythm of creation, when we take time to reflect on creation? Honoring the Sabbath is not part of the "law" and not one of the 10 suggestions – it's the fourth commandment! Creation, itself, has a rhythm. Staying in tune to our personal rhythms, the rhythm of life and creation, all have profound effects on the aging process!

Our lifestyle, including exercise, diet, and maintenance of circadian rhythms, all influence aging, in part, because they turn certain genes on and off. Likewise, Gassen et al., (2016), presented evidence suggesting **life stressors may alter the epigenetics of aging**. Environment and life stressors influence genetic activity. More important, is your **thinking** about your environment and stressors. Can the type of thoughts we have, our thinking patterns, affect our genetic expression and influence the aging process? Thoughts are very powerful. I've shown, in previous chapters, how our thinking "software" can change the "hardware" of our brain. I've also shown how thoughts can modify our experience of pain. Can our thoughts actually accelerate or slow the aging process?

Are some thoughts epigenetically conducive to healthy aging, while other thoughts more conducive to death? **Yes, there's evidence to suggest the quality of your thinking, does influence the genetic expression of aging.** It's not just that bad things happen, and the stress from it ages you; more importantly, it's your thinking about these life events. Zannas and West (2014) showed "exposure to psychosocial stressors can induce lasting epigenetic modifications that carry the potential to shape stress responses." Bad **responses** to stress can epigenetically determine another; likewise, productive **responses** to stress can determine another productive response. How we react to stress can, epigenetically, affect our brains ability to react to stress; the entire process, ultimately, influences aging.

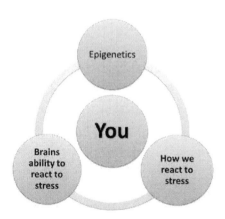

Once again, we see a vicious cycle, this time leading to healthy vs. unhealthy aging. The things we chose to think about can influence the genetically determined aging process. Just as it did in mental health and pain tolerance, this begs the question, "what are the best things to think about, which, has the best effect on our epigenetically determined aging process"?

The bible speaks of generational "curses." Ancient man didn't understand epigenetics; however, they could see certain, less functional, characteristics passed down from generation to generation. Whether you want to call this a generational curse or epigenetics, the fact is, we can have some control over the expression of our genes. If you feel you've been dealt a bad genetic hand, or if it seems your extended family carries certain bad genes – don't worry, there's hope! The information I've shared suggests diet, exercise, maintenance of life rhythms, even correct thinking can turn things around in your life, and the lives of your offspring - you can change the genetic hand your family has been dealt!

Dr. John Kelly, founding president of the American College of Lifestyle Medicine (A.C.L.M.) agrees, "Our lifestyle choices for good or for bad are passed on to future generations." Some of us are a victim of the bad lifestyle choices of past generations. Maybe you have a learning problem or a metabolic health problem you may consider genetic – I wonder if you want to turn some of those genes around – not only for yourself but also for your offspring?

Dr. Kelly says, in the Complete Health Improvement Program (CHIP), "Epigenetics is proving we have some responsibility for the integrity of our genome" (our genes). He summarizes:

> **Changing** your diet and lifestyle…
> changes your epigenome switch settings.
> **Changing** your switch settings…
> changes gene expression.
> **Changing** gene expression
> changes you – literally

It all starts with lifestyle – not just what you **do** but **who** you are!

Does this seem like theory, just conjecture? Can diet, exercise, life rhythms, stress management and correct thinking change your genetic expression, the way your genes are turned on and off? What kind of scientific proof exits in the real world? Let's look at one final researcher, who showed how lifestyle changes can influence cancer genes and melt away hardening of the arteries. Dr. Dean Ornish really brings home the importance of complete lifestyle changes: physically, mentally, and spiritually.

Prostate cancer is a reality for many men. It turns out **some** prostate cancers, found early, can just be observed without any treatment. Dean Ornish et al., (2008) enrolled 30 men with prostate cancer, who were "watching and waiting" before treatment. These men all had prostate biopsies. The DNA, cancer messengers, were examined in the biopsy specimens. These messengers tell us about cancerous gene activity. The 30 men all agreed to intensive lifestyle management for just 3 months. Only 10% of calories from fat (they were on a plant based diet – whole foods), walking at least 30 minutes a day for 6 days a week, stress management 60 minutes a day, and one hour group support sessions a week.

After three months, another round of prostate biopsies showed those cancer gene messengers were all reduced. In fact, the researchers suggest numerous studies have shown "lifestyle changes may modify the progression of prostate cancer" and "healthy diet and lifestyle practices improve recurrence-free and overall survival in colon cancer and breast cancer."

Dr. Ornish was also involved in the famous *Lifestyle Heart Trial* (Ornish et al., 1990). In this amazing study, researchers looked at 48 people who had angiographically proven advanced coronary artery disease. 28 of the participants underwent extensive lifestyle modifications and 20 were assigned to the "usual-care" group. After one year, they performed another round of heart catheterizations which showed the arterial blockages shrank in the group with lifestyle modifications, while the arterial blockages in the "usual care" group worsened.

What happened to this experimental group to improve

hardening of their arteries? **The experimental group were:**

1) On a low-fat vegetarian **diet**: fruits, vegetables, grains, legumes, and soybean products without caloric restriction. They ate as much as they want but no animal products were allowed, except, egg white and one cup per day of a non-fat milk or yoghurt (~10% of calories as fat, 15-20% protein, and 70-75% complex carbohydrates). No cholesterol medications were even used in the lifestyle group!

2) Moderate **exercise** – typically walking 3 hours a week

3) **Smoking** cessation

4) **Stress** management training for one hour a day – stretching, breathing techniques, meditation, progressive relaxation, and mental imagery. All to increase the persons sense of relaxation, concentration, and awareness.

5) Twice a week discussions were held to provide **social support** – to improve adherence to the program, communication skills, and expression of feelings about relationships at work and at home.

Ornish went on to follow 20 of the 28 lifestyle patients for 5 more years and they continued to show improvement of plaques by 7.9%, whereas, the control group continued to worsen by 27.7%. Interestingly, unlike the lifestyle group, half of the control group were on cholesterol reducing medications.

We've seen how diet and exercise work together. The *Lifestyle Heart Trial* also included stress management and social support; more than just diet and exercise, the heart trial was about **lifestyle – it was who they were**! Both the prostate cancer group and the heart trial included an hour a day of stress management. We only have about 18 waking hours a day and half of those are often spent working. That one hour of stress reduction is valuable; for me, it looks like bible study and prayer – an hour long, daily time of renewal. The prostate cancer study had one hour a week group support sessions and the heart trial had twice a week discussions: social support to help with adherence to the lifestyle, communication skills, and expression of feelings about relationships at work and at home. Social support is extremely important, not only when we introduce lifestyle changes, but also to maintain them! Where can we find top quality social support, in an average community? In real life, this looks like a well-functioning church, which values body, mind, and spirit.

So far, we've looked at several theories of aging: metabolic problems such as insulin and sugar metabolism, we also looked at oxidative stress, and finally, at genetic causes of aging; including the hope of epigenetics & lifestyle, to counter this genetic aging process. I would like to share two final theories of aging.

Why do we age? Because the world is aging and we're part of it. We only need to look around us to see the world is decaying. The concept of entropy, the 2nd law of thermodynamics, suggests things always tend toward disorder. 1 John 2:17 says the world is *passing away*, 1 Corinthians 7:31 says the world is *passing away*. Then, Ephesians 2:1-5 suggests when we walk according to the course of this world – we too are *passing away*. However, when we come together in Christ, "by **grace" (graceful aging)**, we can step outside the course of this world. Christ impacts our lifestyle. If there's only one thing you take away from this entire book, please understand, we cannot just pick certain lifestyle components to work on (such a diet or exercise); lasting transformation needs to become a **lifestyle** (who you are). To step out of this dying world, we need to look at the eternal (non-dying) lifestyle of God: the Derek of God.

DEREK: THE **LIFESTYLE** OF GOD

The bible talks about an everlasting "lifestyle" or "way." The word **"way"** in Hebrew is "derek" and refers to lifestyle (Motyer, 2005). A proleptic lifestyle, takes hold of certain aspects of our eternal life even now! Thus, we can echo King David, "lead me in the everlasting way *(derek)*" Psalm 139:24. The writer of Psalms 119 pleads "give me life in your **ways**." *Derek* refers to a way of living, a way of thinking, feeling, deciding; in short, who you are. More importantly, it has to do with choosing Gods lifestyle, His way, His *Derek*.

The lifestyle choices we make always need to be made in the light of eternity! We preserve our lives by having components of everlasting life even today. Derek is the lifestyle of God, the everlasting lifestyle; an everlasting lifestyle which slows the aging process! Why? Because it's everlasting, it's eternal, and we can grab hold of aspects of that eternal life. The eternal ageless lifestyle of God slows the aging process, not just by reducing bad habits and developing good ones; it even modifies our genes; this eternal lifestyle becomes who we are!

Greek philosophers, even before our epigenetic research, understood this transformational effect. The Jewish cultural historian, Craig Keener (1993, p 498), wrote "Greek philosophers spoke of being transformed toward divinity by contemplating divine things." The Apostle Paul said, when we gaze upon God, when we gaze upon Jesus, we are transformed, like gazing into a mirror, we become that reflection.

The immediate followers of Jesus understood the importance of lifestyle and even defined their movement as 'The Way'. Christianity was not something they did, but, who they were! Many contemporary churches are now considering themselves '**Decision-Journey** Churches'. In referring to this type of Christian life, Elmer Towns et al., (2007, p199) says, "To them, belief was a *lifestyle* response, rather than a point-of-crisis decision." 'The Way' is a **decision** which leads to a **journey**. Again Towns (p213) writes,

Too many Christians have reduced the gospel to a certain prayer to pray and a card to fill out. It is unimaginable that the early Christians lived in this manner. Instead, they became followers of "the way" (Acts 9:2) by joining with other people on the same path. In Luke 14, when large crowds were following Jesus, He turned to them and told them that it was not easy and they needed to count the cost before deciding to follow Him.

Followers of The Way, "live, eat and sleep" Christ Jesus. The Way becomes who you are![12]

Lifestyle is never about where you are, but, has to do with a journey from your **limited lifestyle to Gods eternal lifestyle**! The bible calls the turning point "**repentance.**" As we journey with the Lord we continually receive instruction from God, "Whether you turn to the right or to the left, your ears will hear a voice behind you, saying, 'This is the **way** (*derek*); walk in it'" (Isaiah 30:21). If we're sensitive to Gods leading we can hear Him say, "This is My lifestyle; walk in it"!

Repentance, changing the road you're on, has to do with an earnest desire for change! Developing a godly lifestyle, requires we approach it with eagerness. The Apostle Paul writes, "See what this godly sorrow has produced in you: what **earnestness,** what **eagerness** to clear yourselves, what indignation, what alarm, what longing, what concern, what readiness to see justice done" (2 Corinthians 7:10-11). When we develop a "godly sorrow" for our way (our limited lifestyle), our **conscience** increases; as the conflict resolves, our **consciousness** increases (our awareness) and we develop strength to change, an "earnestness and eagerness": *Healing the Heart from the Inside Out*!

---

[12] *Way*, as used in Acts 9:2, is translated in the Greek as *hodos* but as *derek* in the Hebrew (compare Isaiah 40:3 & Matthew 3:3 – the same statement but different translation).

DAMAGE CONTROL

What about those of us who have already succumb to disease? Maybe you've already developed heart disease, cancer, or crippling arthritis; let's face it none of us are getting out of here alive. Is there any damage control possible? Yes, thank God, if there is breath in our bodies, there is hope!

I would suggest, **one last theory of aging**. Many have heard the saying "we must die to live." Aging becomes the way "mortal may be swallowed up by life" (2 Corinthians 5:4). Our body tissues progressively age & decay, and ultimately die, so Christ may become progressively alive in us! 2 Corinthians 4:11, 12a & 16 says,

> For we who live are constantly being given over to
> death...that the life of Jesus may also be manifest in
> our mortal body. So death works in us...Therefore
> we do not lose heart, but though our outer man is
> decaying, yet our inner man is being renewed day by
> day.

Aging is the way "mortal may be swallowed up by life"! In fact, Paul goes on suggesting he prefers to be absent from the body that he may be present with the Lord.

Unless the Lord takes us home at a young age, we'll all experience the eventual decay of our bodies. For some, the 'outward wasting away' will ravage them for years, for others, maybe not so long. 2 Corinthians 4:16 reminds us not to "lose heart" as our spirit can be renewed day by day. No matter where you are in life's journey, you can apply some "damage control."

The lives of many people have become nothing more than treating disease: living from one doctor's appointment to another, one lab & x-ray to another and one painful procedure after another. Instead of preventing disease they've succumbed to it. Sometimes disease is thrust upon us and there was nothing anyone could have done to prevent it, but regardless of the cause, there's hope even for those who suffer a multitude of disease. Psalm 139:8 says, "If I go up to the heavens, you are there, if I make my bed in the depths (or the grave). You are there." No matter what your lot in life, you can always depend on and "hug into Jesus" for help and hope!

MOVING FROM PRINCIPLE TO PRAXIS

You'll recall Jane Vella suggests praxis is 'action with reflection'. Reflection is a key component in transformation. Reflection is taking time to think about an experience; understanding how an experience impacts us and our previously held beliefs and values. "The outcome of reflection is to gain deeper insights that lead to action" (Merriam, 2007, p173). Reflection is the metacognitive (spiritual) experience we've developed throughout this book. Reflective **practice** is how we go about this process of reflection. Prayer is one of our most important reflective practices. Prayer is the ultimate time of reflection as it builds the scaffolding we climb on to objectively look back on ourselves and our life. There, in the arms of prayer, we're whisked away to a place beyond ourselves.

Healing the Heart from the Inside Out: developing our metaphorical heart, to heal our physical heart and lives, requires the prevention and treatment of "heart failure." Dr. Lineaweaver gives us the complete definition of heart failure, "Failure of systemic perfusion, compassion, or **courage** consequent to the default of the heart or one of its metaphorical functions." Aging does take **courage**. Thankfully, God gives us provisions for the journey – garments of salvation!

God provides "Garments of Salvation" to help us along the path of life, along 'the way'; they help us develop a lifestyle which slows the aging process, allowing us to age gracefully. "I will greatly rejoice in the LORD, My soul shall be joyful in my God; For He has clothed me with the **garments of salvation**, He has covered me with the robe of righteousness" (Isaiah 61:10 emphasis added). Jesus not only covered us with the robe of Himself, His righteousness, but also gave us other garments, allowing us to "ride on the heights of the earth." God provides us with garments for healthy living.

Like clothes given to us, these garments may not be your style and may look a little awkward. When you first try them on, they may feel uncomfortable, and not seem to fit. However, rest assured, these garments, or disciplines, are beautiful and fit you perfect! Your old tattered garments are aging you, it's time to put them away. Aging challenges us so we need to develop these disciplines "before the days of trouble come"; however, they're also helpful as "the years approach when you will say, 'I find no pleasure in them'."

Spiritual Disciplines

Spiritual disciplines strengthen us to avoid harmful habits and develop healthy new ones. They help us develop self-control and healthy relationships, allowing us to be highly functional at home and work.

1) Prayer – Ultimately, life itself is a stage allowing us to communicate with God in various ways. God can sometimes seem distant and silent, until we develop a prayer life, allowing us to "hear" Him clearly, and without doubt! However, developing the discipline of prayer takes commitment. You may need to rearrange priorities: get up an hour earlier or go to bed an hour later; regardless of the cost, dedicating time each day, doing business with God and reflecting on the events of our life, is the **most precious thing in life**! What comes to mind when you hear the word "prayer"? E.M Bounds say, "Our short prayers owe their point and efficiency to the long ones that have preceded them" (Earley, 2008, p31). These longer, preceded prayers are a scheduled appointment with God; in a designated time and place, away from distractions. During my dedicated prayer time, I may be found pacing, sitting, kneeling, or on my face before the Creator; always, conversing aloud with God as a friend. Interesting, how often it requires an hour to "take care of business." Christians through the centuries have referred to this

"sweet hour of prayer", in reference to the Garden of Gethsemane; when Jesus suggested His disciples couldn't stay awake for an hour with Him in prayer.

2) Bible Study – How can we expects to walk the "Way", the lifestyle of God, and neglect reading the Bible daily for direction? Having the word of God going through your mind every day is critical and truly healing to your brain and body! Although 'devotionals' have a place in study, it's important to read the bible itself, one "book" at a time. Devotionals only give us the author's **insight**; I want **enlightenment** from God! Therefore, I'm afraid devotionals could actually "quench the spirit." As we systematically read the bible, the Holy Spirit gives us divine illumination; we don't want devotionals leading us in a potentially different direction. Likewise, commentaries should only be used as a resource to understand a confusing passage. According to Robert Sandin (1987) St Augustine,

> allowed the interpreter considerable liberty in reading a '**scriptural** interpretation' into the text. The interpreter may choose to accept any meaning that is 'congruous with the truth taught in other passages of the Holy Scriptures,' even if that particular meaning was not clearly intended by the one who wrote the passage. Indeed, a variety of interpretations only contributes to the richness of the meaning of a biblical passage.

Augustine isn't suggesting a reckless use of the Word of God, he's simply allowing the individual to apply the Word to their lives. Let the Word of God speak to you, don't be afraid of it. At first, you may read several paragraphs, not really understanding all of it; then suddenly, a verse comes forth: behold, God speaks to you! If you do have a difficult time understanding a particular text meet with your pastor or spiritual teacher and they will help you work through it.

Also, your pastor can suggest a particular bible version appropriate for you and an easy to read commentary or dictionary.

3) Memorizing Scripture – The best example of a spiritual reality becoming a physical reality (moving from principle to praxis), is found in the book of John, where the "Word became flesh and dwelt among us." Memorization allows the Word to once again "become flesh." Memorization changes your brain, as stable neurologic pathways are developed. As you memorize scripture your brain becomes the Word of God; as it did with Jesus, the Word becomes flesh! My overall power for living improved dramatically when I began introducing memorized scripture into prayer. It's awesome to have the ability to **claim** promises and **proclaim** blessings exactly as they're found in scripture! Memorization is a skill which requires practice. I find it easier to memorize passages from newer bible translations and begin by memorizing one of the psalms which are very visual. Memorizing scripture also slows memory loss, which declines with age!

4) Church Involvement – Do you have to go to church to be a Christian? Well, maybe not, but if you want to be joyful, you need to spend time with other believers! Healthy relationships with other Christians are extremely important. You'll drown in the sea of other relationships, and life, if you don't have the life preserver we call the church. God ordained certain men and women to lead us through the struggles in life: your pastor is your shepherd, your spiritual leader, and friend. We flourish in the courts of life when we're "planted in the house of the LORD" (Psalm 92:13).

5) Fasting – Spiritual disciplines, especially fasting, requires time to develop but have an amazing influence on your journey. Fasting separates yourself from the world! More importantly, fasting is a "date" with God, a time set aside just for Him. We're reviewing ways to increase your spirit, allow you to overcome bad

habits and develop good ones. Referring to the spiritual discipline of fasting, Isaiah 58:11 says, "and the LORD will continually guide you, and satisfy your desire in scorched places, and give strength to your bones; and you will be like a watered garden, and like a spring of water whose waters do not fail." I always walk away from a fast with new enlightenment and a blessing from the Lord!

6) Honoring the Sabbath – Like fasting, the Saturday Sabbath is a special time reserved for God, and, a well needed day of rest. Sabbath is a time set apart to reflect on God's creation, our personal re-creation, and the deliverance of His people! Psalms 92 tells us we are anointed with fresh oil during the Sabbath and, those who remember the Sabbath, will still bear fruit in old age!

7) Work - Are you understanding how a complete lifestyle develops and how the Kingdom of God becomes who you are and not just what you do? The fourth commandment not only talks about remembering the Sabbath rest but also reminds us to work six days! Work gives us purpose and a sense of accomplishment. Work challenges us, grows us, and keeps us out of trouble, also, work keeps us away from the refrigerator and television. If you don't work, your new job will be getting labs and x-rays done and your appointments are now with the doctor and hospital. It's interesting how God placed the six days of work in the commandment of rest. If your struggling with the six days of work, try honoring the Saturday Sabbath and see what happens!

8) Study – History is moving forward along a purposeful path: God, through the discipline of study and reflection, reveals new insights along the way, not new scriptural/biblical information, but new insights none the less. Richard Foster in his classic book, *The Celebration of Discipline* (1988) writes: "The purpose of the Spiritual Disciplines is the transformation of the person. They aim at replacing old destructive habits of thought with new life-giving habits. Nowhere is this purpose more clearly seen than in the

Discipline of study."

Fosters book reveals, in detail, what spiritual disciplines we need. It's my hope and prayer, this book will teach us how to attain these disciplines. Vemuri et al., (2014) suggested, "Lifetime intellectual enrichment might delay the onset of cognitive impairment and be used as a successful preventive intervention to reduce the impending dementia epidemic." Ask your pastor for good reading material, join training and development programs, even take on continuing college level classes.

9) Exercise – I'll not belabor this point further; through this entire book, I've stressed the integration of body and spirit. Our bodies are just as holy to God as our spirit, and **exercise is another spiritual discipline**. Exercise is a form of praise, a way of saying to God, "Look daddy. See what I can do. Thank-you for my life and my health"!

10) Diet – "You are what you eat"! I've heard this saying many times, but is it true? If you eat animal fat, do you literally become animal fat? Humans do store adipose tissue (fat) in the same way as animals (as animal fat). Truly, we do become animal fat if we eat it! Our **soul** is saved by faith, through grace, and not by following rules; we are arrayed in a robe of Christ's righteousness. However, our day to day **lives** require other 'garments of salvation,' including the garment of a proper diet. We don't earn our way into heaven but we honor the **life** God gave us when we eat correctly. We require a proper diet to live properly.

11) Praise - Isaiah 61 suggests Jesus bestows on us a "garment of praise instead of a spirit of despair." I've defined "spirit" as the content of our thinking. The prophet Isaiah clearly tells us the content of our thinking needs to include praise to the Most High God! Praise is the only correct response a creature can give to the creator and sustainer of the universe!

"THERE BUT FOR THE GRACE OF GOD GO I"

As we were caring for our nursing home patients, I overheard an experienced nurse, Jan Meyer, say, "There but for the grace of God go I." I've since learned this phrase is attributed the English martyr John Bradford. It's said,

> The pious Martyr Bradford, when he saw a poor criminal led to execution, exclaimed, 'there, but for the grace of God, goes John Bradford'. He knew that the same evil principles were in his own heart which had brought the criminal to that shameful end.[13]

Likewise, Jan and I, as we saw the ravages of aging, would proclaim, "There but for the grace of God go I." Thus, the reason for titling this chapter "Graceful Aging." Ultimately, the only hope we have is to depend upon the grace of God. Let us all come humbly and beseech God for grace and mercy. Let us all join in with Bartimaeus, the blind beggar, "Jesus, Son of David, have mercy on me!" Mark 10:47.

---

[13]*A treatise on prayer* by Edward Bickersteth (1822)

CONCLUSION

When anyone hears the word of the **kingdom**, and does not
understand it, the evil one comes and snatches away what
has been sown in his **heart**. Jesus

I've delivered a revolutionary view of human nature by
redefining the word 'mind' and emphasizing our moral nature, using
the word 'heart'. **Magnanimous singularity** seems to best describe
this paradigm, as it unfolds in the lives of those who follow Jesus.

Merriam-Webster Dictionary defines **magnanimous** as,
"showing or suggesting a lofty and courageous spirit." I've tried to
take spirituality out of the hand of mystics and theologians, placing
it properly in the hands of common people, by defining spirit as a
higher level of thinking, which doesn't degrade spirit, but lifts the
importance of our thinking into the heavenly realms, where it should
be. Jesus gave us the Kingdom of God to structure this, otherwise
ill-defined, nebulous spiritual existence. The Kingdom of God, as
applied to our lives, is certainly lofty and courageous, and therefore,
magnanimous!

Paraphrasing Webster's Dictionary, **singularity** is, "One person
– a unit and not dual; peculiar – not customary or usual; the state or
quality of being extraordinary, someone of remarkable character."
Singularity defines the individual unity we should have; not
separating body from spirit. Spirit and body are not dual, rather,
interrelated through 'mind'; both requiring care and nurturing for
survival. Next, as the definition would suggest, Christians are a
peculiar people; an increasingly important characteristic "because
of the increase in wickedness." Christians are peculiar because of
holiness not handicap: we are set apart "for Gods own possession."
Finally, we're not just different, rather, extraordinarily different.
Followers of "the way" develop remarkable character which
overcomes mental illness, and pain, also, guides us into disease

prevention and graceful aging. Followers of Jesus are a **magnanimous singularity**.

Praxis is the application of this magnanimous singularity. With practical application, much of what is now defined as <u>mental illness</u>, melts into imagination, emotional experience, and unstructured thinking. <u>Physical pain</u> is reduced by prevention, and tolerated by understanding, disentangling, and dissociation. The natural <u>aging</u> and decay of our body, is balanced by the increasing growth and renewal of our spirits. Diet, exercise, and disease prevention are natural outflows of a new born-again life. "Whether you turn to the right or to the left, your ears will hear a voice behind you, saying, 'This is the **way (derek)**; walk in it.'" If we're sensitive to Gods leading we can hear Him say, "This is the My lifestyle; walk in it"!
7/3/2017

APPENDIX 1

FOR THE ATHEIST AND AGNOSTIC

Throughout this book, God is referenced as living and intimately interactive with man. Ultimately, God can only be approached by faith but understanding always follows.[14] To help conceptualize the existence of God, this appendix is divided into three sections. First, my personal experience, as the best proof of God comes from an examined life (*The Living of Life Reveals God*). For those who remain skeptical, philosophical and theological proofs follow (*The Thinking about Life Reveals God*). I conclude with a section called "The Numinous" (*The Numinous Reveals God*).

LIVING OF LIFE REVEALS GOD

"In the morning I will order my prayer to Thee and *eagerly watch*"

Every Wednesday, starting from about age 10, a church bus would wind its way through my neighborhood, stop directly in front of my house, and not leave until I got on. This bus ministry had a profound effect on the course of my life. As I dive into the lives of many broken patients, I quickly discover such life-giving **opportunities to succeed often drove right by**. Many never had a church bus pull up in front of their house. Today, as you read these pages a bus, leading to life, has finally arrived. It's my hope and prayer you will get on board!

Life's Ultimate Question

Mom was prepared to answer the **big question every human will raise** at some point in life. I was about 4 years old when I asked

---

[14] Why do we need to come to God by faith and not by sight? It's faith which held Jesus on the cross (Hebrews 12:2)! When we apply faith we become Christ in the eyes of God, and that's what saves us!

the ultimate and most profound of all questions, "**Where did all this come from**"? Thankfully, mom knew I was referring to creation and was quick to answer, "God." I'm sure my attention span was only a few seconds, however, in the trustfulness of a child, who had no reason to doubt, I was a "giant in the faith" and that moment laid the foundation upon which I placed all life events. As suggested above in "The Maturation of Fear vs Trust", "How embarrassing to live 80 years and near the end say, "I never really gave it much thought."

Don't Miss an Opportunity

"Release Time" was another life changing event. Once a month, 5th graders can leave school for an hour and go to church. I've often wondered why some kids didn't take the opportunity to get out of school. I became a Christian at "Release Time." In a gentle, non-degrading manner, the leaders opened our eyes to a God of power and perfection. To experience His presence, we need the covering and protection of Jesus. When given the opportunity, I left my chair, went to the front of the room, kneeled and invited Jesus into my life. Why didn't the other kids go to Release Time?

Seeing God Through His Guidance

Fast forward to 8th grade. I spent the night before vacation with 3 friends. It was that evening, in Greg's garage, I first tried smoking. God had his hand on my life and made sure I would never hang-out with those boys again. During our vacation, these same three boys broke in and terribly vandalized our home. Every room in the house was destroyed. As we opened each door and walked from room to room, I would read things like "helter skelter" painted on the walls. This was the most frightening experience I'd ever encountered!

As I look back, I can see Gods goodness and direction. This experience of evil prevented me from associating further with these boys at a critical stage of my development. God made quite sure I wouldn't be smoking in Greg's garage again. Everything said and done, I harbor no resentment. In fact, as you will see below, one of the boys invited me back to church a few years later. Could I be misinterpreting some of these events? I certainly did when they occurred. At the time, it looked as if the power of evil and hate overcame goodness.

I began 9th grade living with my grandparent's. Grandpa was dying of cancer and I was there to "help." One day a preacher introduced himself and invited us to church where I was baptized. As I left the church a friend stopped me and said, "Now you can't do anything bad again." This same friend spent several years of his adult life in prison. The point of this appendix is not just certain events but examining a **life** lived? Read on...

Seeing God Through Tragedy

During my last two years of high school, I would awake every morning at 4am and drive over 75 miles delivering donuts. This job provided a lot of time to pray, think, hope and dream about life. I resumed the donut route after my 1st year of college. Russell, my 11year old brother, wanted to spend time with me and agreed to get up every morning and go to work. He was excited about his job, and the opportunity to spend time with his big brother, who was home from college. Unfortunately, I had picked up some bad habits at college, and after a few weeks, wanted to deliver the donuts by myself, so my bad habits wouldn't influence or be discovered by him.

A few weeks after Russell was let go, from his donut job, he was critically injured riding his bicycle. My life was devastated and I felt partially responsible. My already crumbling faith in God was finally shattered. Now, 30 years later, I can clearly see Gods sovereign hand, not a murderous but a loving hand. Quoting Kierkegaard, "Life can only be understood backwards, but it must be lived forwards."

Deciding to See God

I first thought about medical school, in my second year of college. During a psychology class I discovered Sigmund Freud was a neurologist. To understand Freuds theories, I thought to myself, I would need to go to medical school. After class, I walked across the street, to the library, and asked the librarian if she had any books about "how to be a doctor." I walked out of the library a new person. I was now a "premed" student.

Grades suddenly became everything! If I kept up my grades, I could act anyway I wanted, without regards to other people or God. I became desperately lost in self. I was miserable and wanted to die! During my 4th year in medical school, on a pediatric rotation, I carried in two large books wondering which one the instructor wanted me to read. Handing me a bible he said, "This is the only book you need in my office."

I had no interest in God, if He did exist, I had only hatred toward Him. I was miserable and often thought about suicide. However, I did have respect for the bible as a book, so I didn't throw it out. Over several months, I found myself repeatedly moving this bible "out of the way," from one spot in the apartment to another. One night a friend came to visit. I let him sleep on the living room futon, where I usually slept, and I retired to an extra mattress lying on the bedroom floor. Nights were always the worst, and again found myself in a state of misery, wondering if all generations in my family had lived such hopeless lives; were they all depressed? I knew dad was a depressed alcoholic. I thought about my grandparents and suddenly understood the joy and hope they had because of God in their lives. **The moment suddenly became surreal**. As I laid on the mattress, the moon shining through the blinds, that bible happened to be in my vision. God doesn't need scientific proof and no one can prove God didn't exist! Belief in God is a decision we make! Suddenly, I could feel a huge weight, literally, being lifted off me! The next morning I awoke a new person and decided to go back home and visit my family, who I'd been alienating due to my suicidal thoughts.

Seeing God in Relationships

God was moving in my life even before I made the move toward Him: miraculously arranging for my wife and I to meet. Internship was the final hurtle before getting a medical license, but I kept putting off the application process. I struggled through nine years of college, was graduating medical school, the internship spots were all filling quickly, and yet, I couldn't get enough motivation to fill out a stupid application! Finally, I called Bay Medical and asked if it was too late to enroll and if I had to fill out an application. They invited me to visit and would help with the process.

All the while God was miraculously preparing events in my wife Brenda's life. The Osteopathic hospital, where Brenda worked, was in the process of merging with Bay Medical. Against Brenda's will, a friend picked up job applications for them both. Amazingly, Brenda got the job at Bay Medical and yet her friend wasn't hired. Certainly, God brought Brenda and I together at Bay Medical Center, and a cord of three strands is not easily broken: **"And so we know and rely on the love God has for us"** John 4:16.

A Postcard from God

I felt an unmistakable leading, the summer of 2007, to attend Community Church. Pastor Don Galardi understood the importance of scripture memorization; not just verses but chapters of the bible. I decided to take his advice, skimmed through the Psalms, looking for a good chapter to memorize and came across Psalms 91. This Psalm is very comforting and reveals, among other things, angels who guard over us. I had Psalms 91 memorized and moved onto Psalms 92 (A Psalm for the Sabbath) before Christmas that year.

Mother became gravely ill, March 2008, and while she laid dying on a respirator, I tried comforting her by reciting Psalm 91. I came to the part about angels guarding over us, and suddenly remembered how she collected angels, having dozens of figurines in her small apartment. The word of God suddenly became alive and active. Mom passed away that spring. During her funeral service, Pastor DeVore, who had no prior knowledge of my memorization of Psalms 91, preached on a particular psalm, "that literary critics believe is the most beautiful ever written." You guessed it, he preached Psalm 91 at mom's funeral! Suddenly mourning turned into gladness, my head bowed and my hands went up in praise to God. **Mom's funeral turned into a worship service**! Psalms 91 was a sympathy card from God: He was sorry for my loss, reassured me that I was ok, mom was ok and we would ultimately be together again. Please take just a moment and read Psalm 91, as if it were a blessing your mom was reading over you, at the time of her death.

Faith Balloons

I was driving home from hospital rounds, Thursday November 12, 2009, contemplating life: wondering if God was real and then wondering why I could ever doubt. I suddenly seen faith as a helium balloon, soaring in the sky and doubt was a very long, thin string, attached to the balloon. I held onto this string of doubt, which kept me anchored secure in the "reality" of this world. If God was just fantasy, then letting go, soaring into total belief and trust, would be totally letting go of reality. I could soar in the heights of faith, not being afraid of floating away into another world, if I held onto this thin string of doubt, "safely" tethered to the earth. What would happen, I wondered, if I finally let go of doubt, believed in and trusted God? **I came home, shared this vision with my wife Brenda and the next day we found out she had breast cancer.**

Brenda and I previously made arrangements to take a few days off work beginning Friday, November 13, 2009. We planned to leave town, but interestingly, never made any specific arrangements. Brenda's gynecologist discovered a breast lump earlier that month and happened to schedule her mammogram that same Friday morning. I packed, while she got her mammogram done, believing we would leave on our trip afterward. Even before she arrived home, I received a call from the radiologist telling me the mammogram was very suspicious for cancer. I was so thankful to be off work that day, as we consoled one another and planned for a breast biopsy the next morning. The cancer came back positive for estrogen receptors, so we were very thankful Brenda "happened" to stop a medication containing estrogen the fall of 2008.

God will glorify himself in all situations, which occurred during Brenda's breast MRI 11/20/2009. The technician was unable to start her IV; after numerous attempts, Brenda requested her mom, who was in the waiting room, be allowed to come in to pray. As Pat prayed over them, the IV was started the very next attempt!

The time came for Brenda to see the oncologist, who would determine if she would need a simple lumpectomy & radiation or a total mastectomy with chemotherapy. The day before, and even during the drive to the oncologist's office, God was speaking to me about "**truth**." As it would turn out, the oncologist read the report wrong, telling Brenda she would need a mastectomy instead of just a lumpectomy. As we both cried, stumbling out of her office, we trusted God for "**truth**" in the situation and later that same morning discovered the oncologist's mistake.

Brenda surgery for excision of cancer and lymph node dissection was 11/24/2009. During the surgery, Pat and I were in the waiting room and a small child was quite distracting, so we moved into the chapel and prayed aloud for 20-30 minutes. I happened to be taking a class entitled "Prayer and Spiritual Warfare." Suddenly, during our chapel prayer, I seen a vision of rejoicing in the operating room and immediately knew the lymph node pathology report came back cancer free and the surgery was ending. I know the timing was correct as the waiting room light changed to "procedure ended" just after we returned.

Seeing God through His Perfect Timing

I may have some insight into Gods direction but no financial sense what-so-ever. We struggled to save money for college, but just purchasing my son's computer used up all our savings. However, God had his own college fund for us.

One month before the first tuition payment, I attended an evangelism training program and was given a book on budgeting. With this large college expense looming, Brenda and I read the book and made plans to sit down the evening of August 5, 2010 and write out a budget. The prospect terrified us! The morning of August 5th, reading in the book of Mark, Jesus told me to "avoid the three 'thorns' of worry, deceitfulness of riches and the desire for other things" and was also reminded He said, "Don't worry about your life, what you will eat or drink or about your body, what you will wear is not life more important than food and the body more important than cloths." That very afternoon, I received a call from my practice manager. For several years, I had been paying premiums on a life insurance policy, that was supposed to be a practice expense. I would be getting a $5000.00 refund check, which, in addition to other unexpected income, almost exactly matched our need and set us in the right direction for the upcoming years. "God moves in mysterious ways His wonders to perform" (William Cowper).

I could go on and on shouting Gods goodness and direction in my life but I think you get the point. The bus has arrived, welcome aboard! My prayer: "O LORD, your hand is lifted high…Let them see your **zeal for your people**" Isaiah 26:11a.

THINKING ABOUT GOD REVEALS GOD

"It is the glory of God to conceal a matter, But the glory of kings is to search out a matter." Proverbs 25:2

I had just finished doing rounds on a dying patient, when I heard "The Cradle Song" broadcasted over the hospital PA system, signifying a baby was just born. The contrast of death and life was complete. As I peered out the window, I sensed God hiding behind the fluffy white clouds, and I murmured, **"I can seee youuuuu."** Life is full of the "twinkling's" of God's presence, but to see Him, we must first be willing to look for Him.

The bible tells us Peter walked on water with Jesus. The Apostle Peter claims to have witnessed Jesus' life, miracles, death, and resurrection and then writes, "we did not follow cleverly devised stories when we told you about the coming of our Lord Jesus Christ in power, but we were eyewitnesses of his Majesty" (2 Peter 1:16). In fact, Bible writers repeatedly tell us, they are telling us the truth![15] But, are they lying about telling the truth?

To answer this question, we need to examine the overall content and structure of their writings. The books of the Bible feed a person spiritual life like no other material on earth, and could only be written by someone with extreme spiritual understanding. **Authors, with such a gift, could not lie about the things they personally witnessed.** The books of the Bible are such high spiritual writing the authors could never have lied and said things like, "I assure you before God that what I am writing you is no lie" (Galatians 1:20). The bible must be trusted completely or the issue of any legitimate spirituality is over!

---

[15] Luke 1:1-4, John 19:35, John 1:4, John 1:34, John 21:24, 1 John 1:1-3, 1 John 4:14, 1Peter 5:1, 1 Peter 5:12, 1 Thessalonians 2:3, 1 Timothy 2:7 and Acts 10:39

Christians point to numerous Old Testament prophecies concerning Jesus' birth, life, miracles, death and resurrection, written century's before, as further proof Jesus existed and is God! Skeptics may claim Old Testament writers were creating the idea of some upcoming Messiah, some hero, just to satisfy the **need for hope** in their lives. Again, skeptics may say Christians took these bits and pieces, from the Old Testament, and applied them to a character named 'Jesus' and after the fact said, "see how Jesus fulfilled all the prophecy"!

No one can dispute information about a "Messiah" scattered throughout the Old Testament. No one can deny Old Testament stories about an upcoming virgin birth in Bethlehem. No one can doubt stories exist of God freeing the slaves and leading them to the "land flowing with milk and honey." There are stories of God providing manna, the bread of life, stories in the Old Testament about an up and coming King and Kingdom which will never end. What about beloved tales of God, Himself, being a sacrifice for man's sin? Oh, how well these scattered Old Testament puzzle pieces fit together: oh, how beautiful a picture of Christ Jesus they create! Some believe all these tales, Old and New Testament alike, to be lies but look at the picture they create!

I recall walking through the Chicago Institute of Arts, admiring the numerous paintings and sculptures, when suddenly I turned a corner and ran into the painting *Two Sisters (On the Terrace)* by Renoir and stopped. The painting was spectacular: a celebration of spring and youthfulness, the colors vivid and artfully placed! The curators knew of its beauty and placed it in the center of the main hall. I stood spellbound for what seemed like an hour and kept returning to the picture throughout the day, to make sure the experience was real. Yet, this is nothing compared to the beautiful picture of Jesus, pieced together as it were, from the Old Testament: an awesome tapestry of a God that created, loved, and bled for humanity. The **beauty of Jesus** provides proof, in and of itself, for those who take the time to truly appreciate it. No one can dispute the beautiful picture of Jesus! Oh what a beautiful picture these **puzzle pieces** create.

No one put the pieces of the puzzle together like the Apostle Paul and no one can dispute the high spiritual content of his writing. When referring to the 'puzzle pieces' he joined and how easily they came together, Paul a "Pharisee of the Pharisees," could not lie and say, "We do not use deception nor do we distort the word of God, on the contrary by setting forth the truth plainly we commend ourselves to every ones conscience in the sight of God" (2 Corinthians 4). Here, Paul appeals to **your** conscience, to your inner sense of what is right, what is good and bad, and says in effect, "take a moment and see the beauty of this picture, in your heart of hearts, doesn't this picture look like truth"! Be truthful with yourselves. In your heart, deep down, doesn't the idea of God, as portrayed in Christ Jesus, just seem right!

It's been said "**the eye can only see** what the mind can conceive." If we never take time to honestly conceive, even the possibility of God, let alone go on and conceive the implications of that reality, we will never "see" him. It's interesting how Christians wonder why some people cannot see the obvious existence of God. I once asked a new Christian how he "discovered" God, to which he replied, "I woke-up."

God clearly reveals himself in creation. Take, for instance, something like the genetic code. Few genetic scholars deny intelligent design; those who do deny it, often have a moral problem rather than an intellectual one. Educators can sometimes mislead young students. Just because a person has a college degree, doesn't give them special knowledge about **life** itself! Institutions of higher learning are filled with people who simply perceive the universe from a strictly objective, scientific viewpoint; this is not the correct way to view our **experience** of existence. Mankind needs to live life not just study it! As noted above, it's in the living of life we best discover what's real!

Wisdom calls out to God. Intelligence is your ability to acquire knowledge. Knowledge is the stuff you know. Understanding is your ability to manipulate all that knowledge, to view all sides and facets of it. Wisdom is something much more complete. Wisdom is your ability to apply understood knowledge. A person capable of looking truthfully at themselves, and all of life, will put **life, and the living** of it together, apply wisdom, and discover God! God loves to be discovered.

As individuals, we start out with nothing but instinct and must learn the very basics of life. Just a few years ago, each of us were trying to comprehend the basic principle that one object plus another object is two objects. Is it any wonder we have a hard time conceiving the infinite? A man trying to understand God is like the sculpture of King David trying to understand Michelangelo. **The created can never fully conceive the creator!**

I've always been fascinated with life, often asking the question, "what do you think's going on." Many people seem quite content living in a mystery. Many live life, have children, enjoy, suffer and die and never understand "what's going on." Rudolf Otto coined the phrase *Mysterium Tremendum*. This phrase refers to the tremendous mystery: the mystery of life. There's something rather than nothing and that something is miraculous. **There is; I am; and there is a great I Am!**

What do you thinks going on? Really, what's your best guess? Do you think you're magnificent or fallen together? What's your best guess? The story is told of a virtuoso violin player who captured large sums of money for concert performances. One day he played on a street corner. It's said many walked by **oblivious to the magnificent**. Likewise, many walk by the course of their lives oblivious to the magnificence of God. Is it possible, in the vast expanses of time and space, **anything** higher than you could exist? Yet, it's so hard for our little minds to grasp the infinite characteristics of God. **Our greatest doubts** are actually Gods greatest praises! "Such knowledge is too wonderful for me; it is too high, I cannot attain to it" (Psalms 139:6). **God presents himself to man in the form of wonder!**

THE **NUMINOUS** REVEALS GOD

Jesus said, "Therefore I tell you, don't worry about your life, what you will eat or drink; or about your body, what you will wear. Is not **life** more important than food, and the body more important than clothes"? Jesus believed **life** itself is more important than food which sustains it. **Life** amazed Jesus; all the varied activities and qualities of it took second place. On the opposite extreme, are those so carried away by all the activities of living, the miracle of **life** itself, is taken for granite and obscured. Those so fascinated by the activities of life always fall short, and are disappointed, as activities inevitably fail. Yet, those fascinated by **life** never fall short; even when our life dies the fact of **life** remains. The reality of **life** should overwhelm us, so much, everything else takes second place. Even in the face of extreme tragedy, illness, pain, or suffering, **life** itself remains miraculous! Jesus' fascination for **life** would come naturally, as he honored the Sabbath: reflecting on His creation and using the time to distance himself from the affairs of life.

Fear seems to be a primary reason people lose respect for **life**. Preoccupied with fear of losing life's basic necessities, we often miss the value of **life**. Jesus' entire earthy ministry was trying to reassure people; moving them to place more value on **life** itself. He tells his disciples "So do not worry, saying, 'What shall we eat?' or 'What shall we drink?' or 'What shall we wear?' For the pagans run after these things, and your heavenly father knows that you need them. But seek first his <u>kingdom</u> and his righteousness, and all these things will be given to you as well."

Fear can be taken to a more basic level, which everyone deals with at some point: the fear of existence, the fear of being. At some point in development we become aware that "we are," that "we exist." We all come to recognize there is something, rather than nothing, and we are distinct in that somethingness. All but the most dumbfounded should naturally experience a **sense of awe**. There are points in everyone's life, even if for a split second, when we get a sense of awe and wonder, bordering on "fear" (respect). This sense of awe is humbling and fearsome and many repress it: favoring the experiences in life, they begin neglecting the fact of **life**.

Existentialism is a philosophical movement, investigating the mystery and experience of one's own existence. Unfortunately, the ideas of many existentialists show clearly how very logical steps can end up in a very illogical place. For example, Friedrich Nietzsche challenged us to experience life without God. Nietzsche's ideas fueled both Hitler's and Mussolini's movements; ultimately Nietzsche succumbed to mental illness in his middle 40's and remained insane until he died 15 years later. The well-known painting called "The Scream," by Edward Munch, portrays a horrified person on a bridge. The painting "powerfully expresses the artist's anxiety and pessimism, caused by the confusion and loneliness of existence" (Magee, 2001, p.213). The experience of **life** itself is much harder for those who ignore the true existential view, given to us by Jesus (the Author and Perfecter of existence). Jesus was the original "existentialist."

Jesus was adamant his followers respect **life**, as from this vantage point, one can best see God! There are people who awake every day and wonder about **life**. But this wonder doesn't end as we walk out the door; it follows us through our daily activity. This commitment to **life** shows us most clearly the creator of life. It's much harder to see the creator if we are too involved experiencing life; less involved in the wonder of **life** itself.

The Numinous

By experiencing **life** itself, we come to the ***numinous***. Rudolf Otto uses this Latin phase meaning "divine majesty" and applies it to the experience of ***numinous awe***. All world religions begin with a sense of awe. By focusing on the fact of "**life** itself" we have sudden moments of an indefinable experience: something clearly separate (holy-incomprehensible) from us exists.

> One is aware that he or she is in the presence of something, or someone, but the awareness is so primitive as to preclude a clear description of what or who. One thing is certain, however: the experiencer stands in awe of that which he is in the presence (Spiceland, 2005, p848).

Once we've established **life** and the existence of God, even through the experience of numinous awe, we can move forward and correctly answer all life's questions, as **God is the central theme around which all questions revolve**. Understanding these concepts is extremely helpful! There are some who can function without this conception, in certain areas of their life, but I wouldn't suggest it! These principles lead to a life that's very rich, rewarding, and challenging. All things considered, some people still deny God. To those I can shed only one ray of hope – Truth!

APPENDIX 2

FOR THE THEOLOGIAN AND COGNITVE SCIENTIST

"Woe to you, scribes and Pharisees, hypocrites, because you shut off the kingdom of heaven from people; for **you do not enter in yourselves**, nor do you allow those who are entering to go in." Jesus

This appendix contains approximately 6000 words describing human nature, which some may suggest is irrelevant in a "self-help" book. But, remember from chapter one, adult education researcher, Lorraine Zinn, suggested a correlation between beliefs, values and/or attitudes, and human behavior. Then medical educator, Dr. Daniel D. Pratt, writes "Learning is most affected by a learner's self-concept and self-efficacy." Truly, our beliefs do bubble out into behavior. Unfortunately, for many people, underlying beliefs have little value as our society has determined truths are not eternal but transient and relative; constructed by each individual. The lack of any underlying beliefs has bubbled out into poor behavior, and ultimately, into poor health. In chapter one we laid down the framework to understand how the brain & mind functions: the cognitive skeleton. In chapter two, as Ezekiel did in the valley of the dried bones, we watched the muscles and flesh form over the bones, by discussing how to best use and hold together this thinking machine. With that in mind, what follows is a life transforming model of human nature: improved health by understanding self.

Below are proofs for a simple, elegant, and functional cognitive paradigm or doctrine of man model: 'mind' is the interface between brain & spirit; 'spirit' is a world of thought; and, 'heart' is our moral compass. What could be more important than correct thinking? Cognition is what makes us most human and highly valued by God!

Correct thinking is healing and Jesus' introduction of the Kingdom of God, **on earth,** was the introduction of correct thinking, the structuring of our spirit, in fact, spiritual formation! Therefore, our spirit could be thought of as a place or an intellectual environment, in as much as, a Kingdom is a place: the 'Kingdom' of God is a model or a paradigm we place in our spirit, to **structure our thinking place** for health and healing.[16]

A NEW PARADIGM FOR SOUL, SPIRIT, MIND, AND HEART

The Mind Recovery Program

SOUL & SPIRIT

What is man and what are the best terms used to express our multiple experiences and states of consciousness. Modern psychiatrists approach mind/brain from an electrochemical standpoint. Neurologists look at brain centers (nuclei) and pathways. Psychologists sometimes look to the subconscious and developed theories of personality to explain man's behavior. Theologians tend to break man's complex cognitive processes into *thought, emotion and will* in relation to soul and spirit.

The definition of 'soul' is generally agreed upon as 'something you are and not something you possess'. You are a living soul, you do not possess one. Throughout this book, I've defined 'spirit' as a higher level of thinking or metacognition. Christians put a very high value on 'spirit'. Spirit is an eternal godlike concept. However, understanding 'spirit' as a higher level of thinking doesn't degrade spirit, rather **lifts our thinking into the spiritual realms where it should be**! Many of us undervalue our gift of thinking; defining it

---

[16] Proverbs 25:28: *Like* a city that is broken into *and* without walls Is a man who has no control over his spirit.

as worldly and not heavenly! Yet, it's not uncommon for people of various religions to suggest their thinking is being carried away, **even to another realm, another place**! The apostle Paul, in 2 Corinthians 12:2, spoke of a man "caught up to the third heaven." Defining spirit as a higher level of thinking brings spirituality to a level common people can understand and atheists cannot dispute; also preventing the dichotomy which dangerously separates body and spirit.

Just as everyone is created in the image of God and given 'common grace', we all possess a spirit, although for some, quite rudimentary. Anthony Hoekema (1994, p.214) comments on the universal and the 'thinking' nature of spirit,

> Pneuma (spirit) may describe man's **self-awareness** or self-consciousness (1 Cor. 2:11). W.D. Stacey makes the point that Paul does not see *pneuma* as something only regenerated people have: "**All men** have pneuma from birth, but Christian *pneuma,* in fellowship with the Spirit of God, takes on a new character and a new dignity (Rom. 8:10)

Not only do we all possess a spirit, but Hoekema gives 1 Corinthians 2:11 as evidence for the metacognitive nature of spirit: "For who knows a person's **thoughts** except that persons own **spirit** within." Spirit is a higher level of thinking, which allows us to know our thoughts (metacognition) and take every thought captive. Proverbs 20: 27 also suggests the metacognitive aspect of spirit, "The spirit of man is the lamp of the LORD, Searching all the innermost parts of his being."

MIND

I discovered a problem in the way theologians define the words soul, spirit, and heart, in regards to *thought (intellectual), emotion (emotional) and will (volitional).* Wheeler Robinson in *The*

Christian Doctrine of Man (1947, p.16) believes *thought, emotion and will* are part of nephesh (soul): "The psychical usage of nephesh is very varied, and covers all kinds of states of consciousness, even volitional and intellectual, though the emotional strongly predominate." Neil Andersons, *The Bondage Breaker* (2000, p. 47), also places these three under the heading of 'soul'. Anthony Hoekema (1994, p.214) will place these same three processes under the domain of 'heart'; "It is also described as the center and source of the whole inner life of man, with thinking, feeling and volition." M.E. Osterhaven (2005, p1133), places *thought, emotion and will* as part of 'spirit': "It is the seat of rationality, determination… emotions." *Thought, emotion and will* need a correct home, are they in soul, heart, or spirit? The truth is these processes (thought, emotion and will) can be attributed to the physical brain itself.

Thought, emotion and will are categorical terms and speak nothing of content, i.e. what we are actually thinking, feeling or what we choose to do. Brain cell firing patterns create the capacity for *thought, emotion and will* but not the actual content. *Thought, emotion and will* are found in brain cell firing patterns which come together to create **mind**. The gestalt of brain cell firing patterns result in the **ability** for the wondrous 'spiritual' world of ideas, which are completely immaterial (nonphysical), and not based on individual brain cell function. Brain creates something above and beyond itself: brain creates the **organ of mind**, an area of potential *thought, emotion and will* which are capable of *ideas, feelings, and desire.* You cannot reduce something to brain which is built in the tool of mind. "Reductionism has been the most powerful explanatory tool in human history; however, it may have met its match in the human mind" (McLaren, 2010, p727).

One might say, "Well of course our brain creates our mind, this is nothing new." God is relaying to us, that our human brain is much more wondrous than we ever believed. Our brain creates this organ of 'mind' which gives the capacity for a spiritual world independent of the brain itself. Mind could be thought of as an 'organ', created by the brain. The physiology (function) of this organ, we call 'mind', is our 'spirit.' Ideas expand, develop upon themselves, and grow to form **a new life (spirit). Therefore, thoughts are freed from the any physical connections, as they are the product of 'mind' not brain!** Our unbelievably complex cerebral cortex is creating a new environment; an area of thought capability: because the actual thoughts do not lie in the brain itself, but above it, <u>**we've now developed a spiritual world**</u>; a spiritual world, even an atheist couldn't deny.

The effects of psychoactive medications, which are physical and influence the brain, prove this point very well. While psychotropic medications are helpful in mental illness they only work in very general, categorical ways, not at the level of changing specific thoughts. Many drugs just slow the brain down in a nonspecific and general way. Benzodiazepines, for example, are not selective at all, as they affect GABA, "the major inhibitory neurotransmitter and it operates in more than a third of CNS synapses" (McCarroll, 2011 Congdon Lecture Series).   People under the influence of antidepressants are less concerned about their distressing issues; but now, many patients tell me, no longer care about anything, including the things they want to care about. Psychotropic medications work at the brain level, in general nonspecific ways, indicating brain neurochemistry only creates the general capacity for thought and not specifics thoughts.

Interestingly, *mind* could be thought of as a unique area, filling the gap between the material world (*brain*) and the immaterial world (*spirit*). **Mind, at the same time, is a physical and spiritual organ** as it's created by the brain (material) but houses the spirit (immaterial). Mind is composed of brain cell firing patterns, yet at the same time, houses the spiritual world of thought.

This theory came to me after reading the March 2005 *National Geographic* magazine. The feature article begins with, "the *mind* is what the brain does." In a time of prayer, it occurred to me the *mind*, as used by the magazine author, might be different than *thought*.

Although the *National Geographic* author (James Shreeve) simply suggests the "brain creates thought", I interpreted this as "brain creates mind, which creates thought." "The mind is what the brain does" but "thought is what the mind does." Brain is creating something distinct from thought: the brain is actually creating an area called *mind*. But what is this thing we call *mind*? There were too many words with the same meaning; thought, cognition, mind and now I was adding spirit to the synonyms.

Ephesians 4:23 refers to the "spirit of the mind."[17] The New Testament word 'mind' is used to translate the Greek words nous and phroneo. Much has been written on this subject, but these two words can be easily distinguished by remembering "nous" as a noun and "phroneo" as a verb. **Truly "mind" is the magnificent combining of noun & verb!** *Mind* is your brain (noun) and, at the same time, your thoughts (verb) but is not just brain or thought. The astute reader maybe discerning Jesus in this whole paradigm: Jesus having both spiritual and physical characteristics, the "Word" which became flesh.

The Apostle Paul suggests this paradigm in Romans 12:2, "Do not conform to the *pattern* of this world, but be transformed by the renewing of your *mind*. Then you will be able to test and approve what God's will is—his good, pleasing and perfect will." This verse suggests *patterns* (including brain cell firing patterns created by this world) influence mind, but when *mind* is renewed, it leads to a good and pleasing life. We should not be conformed to the rudimentary brain *patterns* of this world, but we are to develop renewed 'spiritual' *patterns*.

To achieve health, we cannot be simple stimulus and response creatures, devoid of spirit (Jude 1:19).[18] Rather we must understand, renew, and develop our thinking world, our spirit; and thus, our lives! It's interesting how we become physically *conformed* to the

---

[17] "And be renewed in the spirit of your mind;"
[18] ...worldly-minded, devoid of the Spirit

spiritual patterns we hold. Norman Geisler writes,

> there is clearly an **interpenetration** of the soul and body, which befits a form/matter unity. *Interpenetration* means that the soul influences the body *and* vice versa. For example, grief in the soul affects the body, and pain in the body affects the mind. This psychosomatic affiliation indicates not identity but unity (2004, p.67).

This interpenetration occurs through the intermediary of mind. So, beliefs (good or bad, true or false) not only bubble out into behavior but also into our physical being.

Considering this interpenetration, I've challenged the reader, throughout this book, to consider the bigger question, "what thinking, what spirit, is the most productive." What thinking (spirit) best influences our brain. What **ideas, feelings and motives** are the most productive for our lives. Enter the spiritual, present day, Kingdom of God!

We can decide to fill our mind with the spirit of 'Man on Earth' or the 'Kingdom of God'. Satan is content we live in and develop the 'spiritual' patterns of this world, however, he doesn't want us to enter the 'heavenly realms' and develop the true spiritual patterns of the Kingdom of God, placing us in touch with Gods Spirit!

Many struggle with spiritual concepts because it lacks environment. This explains why so many suffer with 'flight of ideas', complaining they cannot control their thoughts and cannot "turn off" their brain at night. Humans require environment to live. If we are to "die" to this world and live in the spirit, then our spirits require a structured environment. "The natural life owes all to Environment, so must the spiritual" (Drummond, 1883, p116). Therefore, we need to build up the environment of the spiritual world; we need to **develop** a spiritual or thinking place. I discuss this in detail below, in the section "A New Paradigm for the Kingdom of God," but first we must complete the doctrine of man.

HEART

I've suggested the content of mind is spirit (a higher level of thinking) but it says nothing about the morality of those thoughts, feelings, or motives. The metaphorical *heart* is the term we should use for the moral and ethical values of our spirit. Certainly, the word heart stands for the center of our lives, physically and mentally, and is often used in emotional terms. However, *Holman Illustrated Bible Dictionary* (Cowen, 2003) writes this about the heart,

> The heart is spoken of in scripture as the center of the
> moral and spiritual life. The conscience, for instance,
> is associated with the heart. In fact, the Hebrew
> language had no word for conscience, so the word
> "heart" was often used to express this concept

Numerous bible verses suggest the moral nature of heart.[19] Job 27:6 uses the word heart and conscience interchangeably in various bible versions. The phase "upright in heart" is used seven times in the psalms. Understanding this helps us on our way, because, when "The law of his God is in his heart; His steps do not slip" Psalms 37:31.

It's clear the old testament word for heart, **Leb**, and the new testament word for heart, **Kardia**, are often used in reference to our conscience. But, a major premise of this book suggests it's our conscience (*heart*) that gives us consciousness; therefore, increasing conscience increases consciousness, giving us perspective, strength, and self-control in our day to day life. Jewish historian Craig Keener (1993, p550) tells us, "In Jewish tradition "wisdom" and "foolishness" had much more to do with morality than they did in pagan thought." As further proofs, in chapter 1, I referred to the works of Freud, Hegel, and the Apostle Paul. Peter clearly tells us

---

[19] Ps 78:72, Proverbs 11:20, 22:11, Isa 51:7, Mark 3:5, 6:52, 7:21, Luke 6:45, Romans 1:21, 1:24, 2:15, 1 Tim 1:5, 2 Tim 2:22, Heb 4:12, 10:22, Jas 4:8

morality leads to knowledge that in turns leads to self-control, "Now for this very reason also, applying all diligence, in your faith supply **moral excellence**, and in your moral excellence, **knowledge**; and in your knowledge, **self-control**, and in your self-control, perseverance, and in your perseverance, godliness" 2 Peter 1:5-6. A pure *heart* will result in pure health! The words conscience and conscious have a similar etymology. Both words stem from 'conscire' (be aware): com- "with" and -scire "to know." Both terms, conscious and conscience, refer to an "internal knowledge" or "knowledge within oneself."

Increasing morality opens our eyes: "The precepts of the LORD are right, rejoicing the heart; The commandment of the LORD is pure, enlightening the eyes" (Psalms 19:8), and "Your commandments make me wiser than my enemies" (Psalms 119:98a). The opposite is also true, decreasing moral standards clouds our thoughts: "to those who are defiled and unbelieving, nothing is pure, but both their mind and their conscience are defiled (Titus 1:15b), and "My iniquities have overtaken me, so that I am not able to see…And my heart has failed me" (Psalms 40:12b). The intellectual St Augustine agrees, "For Augustine there can be no separation of faith from reason, **of purification of the heart** from **illumination of the mind**" (Sandin, 1987, 27).

Healing the Heart from the Inside Out suggests the importance of healing our metaphorical *heart* before our physical heart, and body, can be healed. Heart is the best term to use for the morality of our thinking world. Ephesians 4:17-18 completely captures this entire *Healing the Heart* paradigm,

> So I tell you this, and insist on it in the Lord, that you must no longer live as the Gentiles do, in the futility of their *thinking*. They are darkened in their *understanding* and separated from the life of God because of the *ignorance* that is in them **due to the**

hardening of their *hearts*.

The word *heart* is used with a moral definition (**hardening** of the heart). *Ignorance* is a result of this moral failure, which leads to darkened *understanding* and futile thinking (decreasing conscience diminishes consciousness).

Expanding the deepest part of our nature, our moral heart, expands our consciousness. The values we hold expand or reduce our conscious experience of life. The 1960's was full of futile attempts to expand consciousness. However, their search was in the wrong direction. **Consciousness is expanded not by declining moral values but by enhancing them.** Through Christ and the Kingdom of God, we have a new conscience which leads to an expanded consciousness and healing.

More importantly, God manifests Himself to us in our heart: Jesus affirms this, and the moral definition of heart, in Matthew 5:8, "Blessed are the **pure in heart** for they will see God." The apologist, C.S. Lewis, felt our sense of morality is one of the best evidences for God: "You find out more about God from the Moral Law than from the universe" (Lewis, 1952, p29). Hoekema (1994, p215) echo's this suggesting, it's in the heart where "God bears witness of himself... Kardia (heart) is supremely the center in man to which God turns." Ancient rabbinic texts even give "Searcher of hearts" as a title for God. (Keener, 1993, p431).

In summary, Paul's use of the words *patterns* and *mind* in Romans 12 help us define terms such as mind and spirit (do not conform to the *pattern* of this world, but be transformed by the renewing of your *mind)*. Ephesians 4 defines the word *heart* as the moral aspect of our spirit, and if hardened, results in spiritual (cognitive) decay (the *ignorance* that is in them **due to the hardening of their *hearts***). Today we are in a much better position to properly define man as we have both the Old and New Testaments, improved theology and proper hermeneutics, but also, we have modern psychological models and a much better understanding of neurology and neurochemistry. A standard nomenclature and definition for brain, mind, spirit and heart are essential if these various disciplines are to work together!

The spiritual world is truly a thinking world for those who choose to develop it. It begins as a mustard seed when we are born again and soon like yeast it infiltrates our entire life, physically and mentally. Jesus suggested the Kingdom of God is the best structure for our spirits. Since spirit is best thought of as a place, spiritual formation is the construction of the Kingdom of God in our spirit. However, as we review these spiritual constructs below, let us never forget the ultimate Kingdom is the Kingdom to come!

A NEW PARADIGM FOR THE KINGDOM OF GOD

IMPORTANCE TO JESUS

We need to take a moment to clarify the difference between the 'Kingdom of Heaven' (*basileia ouranos*) and the 'Kingdom of God' (*basileia theos*). Jesus would never use the word 'God' around children, nor would he allow His disciples to use the word 'God' in public; rather the phase Kingdom of Heaven, a circumlocution, would be used in these circumstances. However, when debating with the Pharisee's Jesus would use the term Kingdom of 'God' for emphasis. While the terms are often used interchangeably, Vine's Expository Dictionary suggests "The Apostle Paul often speaks of the Kingdom of God, not dispensationally but morally". Suggesting the kingdom of God is everywhere and above all the dispensations of the kingdom of heaven.

The ministry of Jesus centered around the Kingdom of God. However, even before Jesus started preaching, John the Baptist was preparing people for His Kingdom message: "In those days John the Baptist came, preaching in the wilderness of Judea and saying,

'Repent for the **kingdom of heaven** has come near'" Matt 3:1-2. Preaching the Kingdom of God can be dangerous, "And after John had been taken into custody, Jesus came into Galilee, preaching the gospel of God, and saying, 'The **time is fulfilled**, and the kingdom of God is at hand; repent and believe in the gospel'" Mark 1:14-15.

Christians believe Jesus came to earth to "die for our sins," which is true. However, had we asked Jesus, at least in the beginning of his ministry, he may have had a different agenda. In fact, Jesus said preaching the Kingdom of God was the reason He was sent to earth: "The people were looking for him and when they came to where he was, they tried to keep him from leaving them. But he said, 'I must proclaim the good news of the kingdom of God to the other towns also, because **that is why I was sent**,'" Luke 4:42-43.

Jesus commissioned His apostles to preach the Kingdom of Heaven and made it very clear the Kingdom was to be our message as well: "**As you go**, proclaim this message: 'The kingdom of heaven has come near.' Heal the sick, raise the dead, cleanse those who have leprosy, drive out demons. Freely you have received, freely give," Matt 10:7-8. Even after His death and resurrection Jesus was still speaking about the Kingdom, **"After his suffering**, he presented Himself to them and gave many convincing proofs that he was alive. He appeared to them over a period of 40 days and spoke about the kingdom of God," Acts 1:3. Finally, Jesus said He would not return to earth until information about the Kingdom of God is preached in the whole world: "Because of the increase of wickedness, the love of most will grow cold, but whoever stands firm to the end will be saved. And this gospel of the kingdom will be preached in the whole world as a testimony to all nations, and **then the end will come**," Matthew 24:12-14.

In the next two sections, I'll review two important premises. First, aspects of the Kingdom are actualized, even now, residing in our hearts. Second, our nebulous thinking world (our spirit), is best structured as a kingdom, the Kingdom of God.

KINGDOM OF HEAVEN ON EARTH

When we hear the phrase 'Kingdom of Heaven' many immediately think about heaven itself or the end of time. Theologians use the word **eschatology** when referring to "end times," and in the end, God will set up the ultimate Kingdom of Heaven. This end time perspective is called "consistent eschatology" by Albert Schweitzer (Bruce & Scott, 2005). However, many theologians believe components of the Kingdom of God are here with us now! This belief is call "realized eschatology" by Otto and Dodd (Ibid). Commenting on this realized eschatology is G.E. Ladd (2005, p.659),

> The mystery of the kingdom is this: Before this eschatological consummation, before the destruction of Satan, before the age to come, the kingdom of God has entered this age and invaded the kingdom of Satan in spiritual power to bring to people in advance the blessings of forgiveness (Mark 2:5), life (John3:3), and righteousness (Matt. 5:20; Rom. 14:17), which belong to the age to come. The righteousness of the kingdom is an inner, absolute righteousness (Matt. 5:20, 48) that can be realized only as God gives it to people.

Jesus brought the Kingdom of God to earth, so where is? "Once, having been asked by the Pharisees when the kingdom of God would come, Jesus replied, "The coming of the kingdom of God is not something that can be **observed**, nor will people say, '**Here it is**' or 'There it is,' because the kingdom of God is in your **midst**" Luke 17:20-21. We can draw three important points from this verse. First, because Jesus was standing directly in front of them, and yet, said it is "not something that can be observed," suggests His immediate person, at least in that moment, was not the Kingdom of God. Second, the "realized" Kingdom of God on earth is certainly not a defined place or thing, as again He said, "nor will people say here it is or there it is." However, when Jesus takes his rightful place in our lives, beginning in our 'thinking place" the kingdom of God is "in our midst" even now! Numerous translations of Luke 17:21, follow the King James version saying, "the kingdom of God is **within you**."

Jesus was, and is, so misunderstood: the disciples awaiting Him to overthrow Roman rule and establish His Kingdom; Jewish leaders were appalled, not only by His claims to be Messiah, but also God Himself. Even today, many view Jesus simply as the person who died for their sins. Yes, Jesus died for our sins, but He brought the Kingdom of God to earth: He taught people to think!

Alexander the Great brought Greek culture, including the teaching of Plato, throughout the ancient world. Jesus was raised in Nazareth, near Galilee where Hellenistic (Greek) culture was quite prominent. I'm not suggesting Jesus was a Hellenistic Jew, but He was certainly familiar with this type of thinking. Also, although we have no idea how long Joseph, Mary and Jesus spent in Egypt, one of the largest Jewish communities was located in Alexandra, the cultural center of the time. The Holy family would have been exposed to the well-educated Jewish community residing there. Jesus understood Jewish theology but also Greek thinking.

Certainly, Jesus was very interested in our thinking. In Matthew 5 Jesus teaches the emotion of anger is the real issue not just the acts which follow, such as murder. Lustful thinking is the real issue not just the act of adultery. Jesus said, "The **time is fulfilled**, and the kingdom of God is at hand." Jesus fulfilled not only Jewish prophecy but also Greek philosophy.

Jesus brought aspects of the Kingdom of God to earth and it currently resides in the **"hearts and minds"** of His people! Vine's Expository Dictionary says, "So far as this earth is concerned, where the King is and where His rule is acknowledged, is, first, in the heart of the individual believer." Numerous authors attest to the Kingdom of God in the "hearts" of believers. Stephan Macchia (1999, p37) says, "Now, the kingdom of God does not refer to a geographical territory in which God is King. Instead, it means a condition of the heart and mind and will where God is Lord of all." In his classic work *Rediscovering the Kingdom*, Myles Munroe (2004, p93) says, "The Kingdom of God on Earth is God's rulership within the hearts and spirits of believers." Munroe goes on to say,

> The driving motivation of Jesus' life was not to get us to heaven—that is the goal of 'religion'—but to get heaven to us. Jesus' passion was to establish His Fathers Kingdom *on earth* in the *hearts* of men. (Ibid, p 139)

The Dictionary of TNIV terms (Holy Bible, p1385), defines "Kingdom of God":

> The kingdom of God as Gods special rule in the *hearts* of believers and his gracious restoration of the goodness of the creation was initiated through the coming of Christ and will be consummated when Christ returns to bring His saving work to completion.

Erickson's textbook of *Christian Theology* also suggests the kingdom of God is where God reigns in our hearts,

> To determine the real nature and purpose of Christianity, Rauschenbusch observes, we must see it in its pure and unperverted form as it was in the heart of Jesus Christ, for it has been modified in significant ways throughout church history. Jesus' understanding and expression of Christianity can be summed up in the simple phrase "**the reign of God**." It was the center of his parables and prophecies. It was the basis for all that he did. This is the first and

most essential dogma of the Christian faith. The reign of God is the lost social ideal of Christianity. What Rauschenbusch is calling for is a renewal of Jesus' own spirit and aims. Jesus' teaching regarding the reign of God in **human hearts** was not something novel and unprecedented, according to Rauschenbusch. Rather, he was simply continuing and elaborating the prophets' emphasis on personal and social righteousness. Jesus opposed the popular conceptions at those points where they were in conflict with these ideals. What he proposed was a **kingdom of God on earth**; he never mentioned it in connection with heaven. (2004, p122)

To understand Jesus' thinking about the Kingdom of God it helps to understand a little about the culture of His time. Intertestament Jews thought of the Kingdom of God in the abstract. Julius Scott (2004, p297) writes, "In the Hebrew, Aramaic, and Greek languages the words for "kingdom" are all **abstract.** In the ancient world, "kingdom" referred to lordship, rule, reign, or sovereignty, not primarily to a geographical area." Yet another synonym for the "Kingdom of God" would be the "Sovereignty of God."

In Jesus' last statement about His Kingdom, before His crucifixion, Jesus answered Pilate saying, "My kingdom is not of this world. If My kingdom were of this world, then My servants would be fighting so that I would not be handed over to the Jews; but as it is, My kingdom is not of this **realm**," John 18:36. Concerning this verse Matthew Henry (1961, p1616) writes,

Its nature is not worldly; it is a kingdom within men, set up in their hearts and consciences, its riches spiritual, its powers spiritual, and *all its glory within.* The ministers of state in Christ's kingdom have not *the spirit of the world...* Its guards and supports are not worldly; its weapons are spiritual... Its subjects, though they are in the world, yet *are not of the world;* they *are called and chosen out of the world,* are born from, and bound for, another world; they are neither the world's pupils nor its darlings, neither governed by its wisdom nor enriched with its wealth.... he rules in the minds of men by the power of **truth**..... the spirit and genius, of Christ's kingdom, is truth, divine truth. When he said, *I am the truth,* he said, in effect, I am a king. He conquers by the convincing evidence of truth; he rules by the commanding power of truth, and *in his majesty rides prosperously, because of truth...* The subjects of this kingdom are those that are *of the **truth**.*

Finally, G.E. Ladd (2005, p.659) writes, "The coming of the kingdom of God in humility instead of glory was an utterly new and amazing revelation. Yet, said Jesus, people should not be deceived. Although the present manifestation of the kingdom is in humility—indeed, its Bearer was put to death as a condemned criminal—it is nevertheless the kingdom of God."

THE COGNITIVE KINGDOM

Jesus said, "Your kingdom come. Your will be done, on earth as it is in heaven." Clearly, the Kingdom is where Gods will is done (where God reigns), and individually, is in our hearts and minds! It's interesting how often the Kingdom of God is referred to as a cognitive function. A scribe once answered Jesus **intelligently,** and because he showed *understanding*, Jesus told the scribe, "You are not far from the Kingdom of God," Mark 12:34. The German theologian Albrecht Ritschl, looked at cognitive concepts as a place, suggesting the Kingdom of God is a **realm** of righteousness and ethical values (Erickson, 1998, p.1163). As the Apostle Paul traveled on his missionary journeys his theme was always the Kingdom of God: "And he went into the synagogue and spoke boldly for three months, reasoning and persuading concerning the things of the kingdom of God," Acts 19:8. However, for Paul, the Kingdom was not just a physical place, or even in our physical bodies, but a "place" of values and virtues. "For the kingdom of God is not eating and drinking, but **righteousness and peace and joy** in the Holy Spirit," Romans 14:17.

However, the Kingdom of God, as the phase suggests, is a construct or a place, a Kingdom. The Kingdom of God is a 'Thinking Place': Its cognitive constructs are the best structure for our thinking world. Jesus understood our spirit (our thinking) needs structure and environment so He determined to organize our thinking into a place called the Kingdom of God. Proverbs 25:28 says, **"Like a city that is broken into and without walls Is a man who has no control over his spirit."** The 'city' of our spirit must have walls and structure. Yet we often try to structure the walls of our thinking the way **we** want it; to build up **our** kingdom, with **our** walls of protection, or look to the 'security' of walls found in the kingdoms of man on earth. Isaiah 25: 11b – 26:3 compares the Kingdom of God with the kingdoms of self & man on earth:

> God will bring down their pride despite the cleverness of their hands. He will bring down your *high fortified walls* and lay them low; he will bring them down to the ground, to the very dust. In that day this song will be sung in the land of Judah: We have a **strong city**; God makes salvation its walls and ramparts. Open the gates that the righteous nation may enter, the nation that keeps faith. You will keep in perfect peace him whose mind is steadfast, because he trusts in you.

Here Isaiah is referring to a fortress that can develop in your thinking place, a fortress of pride. Real peace can only be achieved when we enter the gates of Gods Kingdom. One could suggest this refers to the physical walls surrounding Judah and not your thinking place. But, the last verse it says, "You will keep in perfect peace him whose **mind** is steadfast, because he trusts in you." They're in perfect peace because they trust in the walls of Gods Kingdom and His protection.

2 Corinthians 10:3-5 refers to another fortress that can develop in the thinking place of your spirit, "the weapons of our warfare are not of the flesh, but divinely powerful for the destruction of **fortresses**. We are destroying **speculations** and every lofty thing raised up against the **knowledge** of God, and we are taking every **thought** captive to the obedience of Christ." Paul's suggesting **speculations, knowledge** and **thoughts** could be thought of as a fortress; he warns us, this thinking place, could turn into a demonic fortress against God; where speculations, knowledge and thoughts are raised up against Him.

Lucifer was not at all happy when Jesus allowed humans to enter the spiritual realms. Therefore Jesus, referring to the Kingdom of God, suggests we must forcefully "enter it" (Luke 16:16). The book of Ephesians is about activity in the spiritual world, especially about the war going on for this "**heavenly realm**", including your place in it, your "thinking place." The heavenly (thinking) realms are a potentially dangerous place, and it's only "in Christ" that we are safe and blessed in this heavenly realm: "Praise be to the God and Father of our Lord Jesus Christ, who has blessed us **in the heavenly realms** with every spiritual blessing in Christ", Ephesians 1:3.

Thankfully Jesus is seated **in** the Heavenly realms far above any destructive demonic forces.

> I pray also that the **eyes** of your **heart** may be enlightened in order that you may know...his

> incomparably great power for us who believe. That power ... which he exerted in Christ when he raised him from the dead and seated him at his right hand in the **heavenly realms**, far above all rule and authority, power and dominion... Ephesians 1:18-20.

Paul goes on to show how God "raised us up with Christ and seated us with him **in the heavenly realms**" Ephesians 2:6. In fact the word Heavenly realms is used five times in the book of Ephesians; it's here we learn our battle is not against the kingdom of man on earth but against the "spiritual forces of evil in the **heavenly realms**" Ephesians 6:12. Paul understood your spirit to be a place, a place in the heavenly realms!

Jerome Lawrence said, "A neurotic is a man who builds a castle in the air. A psychotic is the man who lives in it. A psychiatrist is the man who collects the rent." This saying is very unfortunate and inaccurate because neurotics and psychotics are not creating (understanding) anything, they're simply responding to life and its circumstances! I'm suggesting the construction of a spiritual Kingdom; one of knowledge, understanding, and truth. Let us not devalue our thinking. A kingdom you will develop: The kingdom of self, the kingdom of man on earth, the kingdom of darkness or the Kingdom of God. Our spiritual, thinking world must have form and structure, why not make it the Kingdom of God!

APPENDIX 3

FOR THE CHILD AT HEART

"I praise you Father, Lord of heaven and earth, because you have hidden these things from the wise and learned, and revealed them to little children." Jesus (Matthew 11:25)

We can't learn anything if we "know it all." A.W. Tozer (1948, p.24) wrote, "Now as always God discovers Himself to 'babes' and hides Himself in thick darkness from the wise and the prudent." The modern age has brought us knowledge at the expense of imagination. Richard Foster (1988, p25) sanctifies our imagination,

> We can descend with the mind into the heart most easily through the imagination...We must not despise this simpler, more humble route into God's presence...God created us with an imagination, and as Lord of his creation he can and does redeem it and use it for the work of the kingdom of God....In fact, the common experience of those who walk with God is one of being *given* images of what can be...God so accommodates, so enfleshes himself into our world that he uses the images we know and understand to teach us about the unseen world of which we know so little and which we find so difficult to understand

The geography of the Holy Land is landscaped in analogy. The bible is full of imagery: Jesus the master of metaphor, parables, symbols, and analogy. Many Old and New Testament concepts come to life as they present analogies about the kingdoms of this world and the Kingdom of God.

The creator of Sherlock Holmes, Arthur Conan Doyle says "I consider that a man's brain originally is like a little empty attic, and you have to stock it with such furniture as you choose." This empty attic is upgraded in the 2012 BBC program where Sherlock says "I need to go to my mind palace." Why not upgrade your mind, even further, into a kingdom, The Kingdom Of God? But what are you going to stock it with? At one point in history God dwelt among men in a tabernacle filled with utensils, each having very significant meanings. God now encamps with us in the spiritual Kingdom of our mind, the Kingdom of God on earth; we're encouraged to fill it with the utensils of His word!

To this end, I provide the story of a character named "Mind." Mind was lost but enters a world, a Kingdom, which rescues him. His story is our story and his developing world needs to be ours. The tools he finds are bible verses I've memorized, developed during prayer, and are rehearsed throughout the course of each day, to bring the Kingdom of God alive! You're welcomed to use the symbols given here, along with their attached bible verses, but I would encourage you to develop your own. One of the enduring legacies of this book is the redefinition of the word 'mind'; to that end, I present, *"Mind was Lost."*

MIND WAS LOST

Mind was lost. The last thing he could remember was the safety and security of his parent's estate. But what happen? There must have been a battle with their rival, The Wills. Mind may have sustained an injury, as he lost all sense of direction: north, south, east and west were lost. Adding to the confusion, Mind acquired the ability for vertical travel. The loss of direction was dizzying as he was floating in disorientation. Mind suspected, he was in the Freeland's: only in Freeland can one move vertically, and what some have called, 'Heart Travel'.

Mind was lost, and disoriented, floating aimless in the 4-dimensional world; desperately in need of stability. Mind felt as if he were falling apart. Heart Travel was new to him and he quickly found himself soaring through the heights of conscience. One after another, Mind kept running into the jagged and sharp cliffs of Guilt and Shame.

Mind was lost. Alone and fearful of invading thoughts. Weeds of Worry began to grow all around, sometimes entangling him, resulting in sudden attacks, out of nowhere, by Panic. Other times, he found himself floating among the thorns of selfish desire and the deceitfulness of riches. This was turning out to be a most hostile environment. Mind often wandered aimlessly along paths of ideas, but they all seemed to lead nowhere: all paths seemed to meander around the garden of confusion.

Mind was lost and ran into yet another problem; pointed Accusations flying about him. The Accusations where sharp and flying everywhere; their impacts were painful, and over time drained him of his strength, but also, of his sense of truth and reality. Occasionally mind could see disc-like Spirit Pods floating above all the hopelessness; impervious to the attacks of Panic, Accusations, the thorns of flesh and those entangling weeds. The Pods also seemed to be in control of Heart Travel.

Mind was lost, alone and suddenly found himself in Darkness. Darkness was the father of all Lies and the keeper of the garden of confusion. Lies were the worst of all Minds adversaries and quickly surrounded him: now in complete Darkness he became a slave to Lies.

Mind was lost in Darkness and paralyzed by Lies. His movement in this 4-dimensional world had stopped: he lost his mind! Thankfully, Truth sensed Minds presence in Freeland: gradually, into Minds pain and stagnation, the Wind of Change began to blow. The Wind carried him, "It seemed to blow where it pleased, he could hear its sound but couldn't tell where it came from or where it is going." The Wind led him to Evangelion who proclaimed loudly "I have good news, Darkness has been defeated." Mind questioned the defeat, as just another lie, because weeds and thorns still surrounded him, and the attacks of Panic and Accusations still raged on. Evangelion reassured Mind that Truth had defeated Darkness and his Lies; it was only the stench which lingered!

Mind was lost: his judgment so clouded and the stench so overpowering, he doubted the 'good news'. Although he doubted, hope began to grow. The more Mind investigated Truth, the more he could see 'Twinklings', a numinous awe. "Twinklings of Insight" started to appear in the heavens; revelations of a King, and Mind began to see the floating Spirit Pods as part of a larger Kingdom. Evangelion told him the Pods of Spirit were the substance and structure Mind so desperately needed. Truth offered Mind his own Spirit Pod, his own Thinking Place; but still, Mind had to climb on board.

Truth provided stairs which helped Mind climb onto the Pod. The first step was called *pride*; Mind had to "cast it down to the ground, to the very dust". The second step was over *shame & disgrace*, as Mind declared, "In You, LORD, I have taken refuse, let me never be put to shame." The next steps, were rising above *anger* (the destroyer), *anhedonia* and *apathy* ("They surrounded me on every side, but in the name of the LORD, I cut them down"). Mind had to the ascend over the steps of *cynicism* and *pessimism* ("All the nations surrounded me, but in the name of the LORD, I cut them down"). Finally, Mind ascended over the steps of *discontent, despondency and total despair* ("They swarmed around me like bees, but they were consumed as quickly as burning thorns; in the name of the LORD, I cut them down"). As Mind climbed aboard, he discovered a wonderful sense of security and wellbeing.

Mind was so lost, and in need of stability, that even his Spirit Pod seemed unstable; floating as it were, above the ground, unsupported in space. He could feel the Pod rocking back and forth, until two large boulders appeared, one on each side, stabilizing the Pod. Engraved on the boulder to his left was the word 'Ebenezer' and Mind agreed, "Thus far the Lord has helped us." This Ebenezer, attesting to the past, was balanced by another large boulder, on the right, holding a rock-solid promise for the future, "Do not fear for I am with you, do not be dismayed for I Am your God, I will strengthen you and help you and uphold you with my righteous right hand."

Mind was lost, but suddenly, in the center of the pod, a small plant began to grow; quickly developing into a large Tree. Mind recognized the Tree; being the same one found in his parent's estate. Mind remembered how the Tree of Spirit comforted him during storms; providing healing, strength, and renewal. As a child, Mind would sometimes get lost in the many gardens, and yet, could always see the tall Tree; giving him a sense of direction and center. As the Tree grew, it provided gifts and nourishing fruit. The Tree promised to scrutinize his path, guide him into all truth and disclose to him what is to come.

Mind was lost, but discovered relief from the painful Accusations. As he climbed into the trusting arms of the Tree, he surveyed the hostile environment and loudly proclaimed, "May those who rage against me surely be ashamed and disgraced but instead of my shame I will rejoice in my inheritance and instead of my disgrace I will receive a double portion."

Mind was lost, still thirsting for Truth, until he discovered a fountain of blessings to drink from; a fountain flowing with peace, "May the God of peace equip you with everything good to accomplish his will and may he work in you what is pleasing to Him." He also found an altar of incense, which burned, filling his life with hope, "May the God of hope fill you with joy and peace as you trust in Him."

Mind was lost as he suddenly found himself drowning. The Pods waterfall of imagination and emotion began to gush forth from behind him, quickly flooding his Pod. At first, Mind panicked but quickly learned to appreciate and control the deluge, discovering it colored and nourished his Pod, making it exciting and beautiful. But, in the wake of such torrent, developed a Mire of Memories and a Babbling Brook of Possibilities. Vapors would occasionally build-up and release from the Mire of Memories; however, Mind simply presented them to Truth. Mind learned to laugh, and even make fun of the Babbling Brook of Possibilities, as he would say, "Declare the things that are going to come afterward, That we may know that you are gods; that we may anxiously look about us and fear together", declaring to the Babbling Brook of Possibilities, "You are less than nothing and can do nothing at all." Living in the present, he gained control; understanding memories are past and possibilities are not Truth. As Mind gained control, he discovered the waterfall, mire, and babbling brook, all joined with the flow of time and events, into the Stream of Consciousness; together they turned the Waterwheel of Activation, which energized his Pod. He learned the waterwheel was more effective if he allowed the stream to flow freely off the Pod; never allowing the tailrace to return and flood the headrace.

Mind was lost. Feet still entangled: Truth provided a Sword to cut the vines of Vane Responsibility. Vision still clouded: Truth provided a Helmet of Clarity to see through the visions and nightmares of failure. Still remembering the Accusations: Truth even took off His own breastplate of righteousness, presenting it to Mind. Still exposed to the flaming arrows of Lies: Mind picked up the Shield of Faith, "You will not be afraid of the arrows that fly by day or the pestilence that stalks at darkness." Finally, being given the Belt of Truth, Mind could see the flaming arrows for what they really were, only paper airplanes.

Mind was lost. Tired, from always standing-up for himself; but suddenly, a seat appeared; the Seat of Favor. "It finds favor, if for the sake of conscious toward God, a man bears up under sorrow when suffering unjustly...if when we do what is right and suffer for it, we patiently endure it, this finds favor with God."

Mind was found! The Winds of Change constantly blew his Pod in endless directions; until one day, Truth provided Mind with a rope, the Rope of Hope. A rope firmly anchored in the Temple of Heaven. As Mind held tightly to the Rope of Hope, Truth safely pulled him through the labyrinth of Freeland.

Mind was found! The Light of knowledge had dispelled the Darkness of ignorance. His Pod began to merge with other Pods;

and finally, all into the Pod of Truth. Mind celebrated as he found himself part of a glorious Kingdom and could finally see Truth clearly.

REFERENCES

Anderson, N. T. (2000). *The Bondage Breaker: Overcoming Negative Thoughts Irrational Feelings Habitual Sins.* Harvest House Publishers.

Artinian, N. T., Fletcher, G. F., Mozaffarian, D., Kris-Etherton, P., Van Horn, L., Lichtenstein, A. H., ... & American Heart Association Prevention Committee of the Council on Cardiovascular Nursing. (2010). Interventions to promote physical activity and dietary lifestyle changes for cardiovascular risk factor reduction in adults a scientific statement from the American Heart Association.*Circulation, 122*(4), 406-441.

Atlas, L. Y., & Wager, T. D. (2012). How expectations shape pain. *Neuroscience letters, 520*(2), 140-148.

Bandura, A., O'leary, A., Taylor, C. B., Gauthier, J., & Gossard, D. (1987). Perceived self-efficacy and pain control: opioid and nonopioid mechanisms. *Journal of personality and social psychology, 53*(3), 563.

Beck, A. T., & Rush, A. J. (1988). Cognitive therapy. In H. I Kaplan & B. J. Sadock (Eds.), *Comprehensive textbook of psychiatry: 5* (pp. 1541-1550). Baltimore: Williams & Wilkins.

Bair, M. J., Robinson, R. L., Katon, W., & Kroenke, K. (2003). Depression and pain comorbidity: a literature review. *Archives of internal medicine,163*(20), 2433-2445.

Blumenthal, J. A., Babyak, M. A., Doraiswamy, P. M., Watkins, L., Hoffman, B. M., Barbour, K. A., ... & Hinderliter, A. (2007). Exercise and pharmacotherapy in the treatment of major depressive disorder.*Psychosomatic medicine, 69*(7),

587.

Bostock, Sophie, Steptoe, Andrew, Association between low
functional health literacy and mortality in older adults:
longitudinal cohort study, *British Medical Journal*, 15,
March 2012; 344:e1602.

Boyd, R., & Myers, J. (1998). Transformative Education.
International Journal of Lifelong Education, 7(4) (October-
December 1988): 261-284.

Bokov, A., Chaudhuri, A., & Richardson, A. (2004). The role of
oxidative damage and stress in aging. *Mechanisms of
ageing and development*, *125*(10), 811-826.

Braskie, M. N., Boyle, C. P., Rajagopalan, P., Gutman, B. A.,
Toga, A. W., Raji, C. A., ... & Thompson, P. M. (2014).
Physical activity, inflammation, and volume of the aging
brain. *Neuroscience*, *273*, 199-209.

Brewer, G. J. (2010). Epigenetic oxidative redox shift (EORS)
theory of aging unifies the free radical and insulin signaling
theories. *Experimental gerontology*, *45*(3), 173-179.

Brown, P. (2000). *Augustine of Hippo: a biography*. Berkeley
California: University of California Press

Brown, S. A., Pagani, L., Cajochen, C., & Eckert, A. (2011).
Systemic and cellular reflections on ageing and the
circadian oscillator–A mini-review. *Gerontology*, *57*(5),
427-434.

Bruce, F.F., & Scott J.J. (2005). Eschatology. *Elwell's Evangelical
Dictionary of Theology (2ⁿᵈ ed.)*. Grand Rapids, Mich.:
Baker Book House.

Bygren, L. O., Kaati, G., & Edvinsson, S. (2001). Longevity

determined by paternal ancestors' nutrition during their slow growth period. *Acta biotheoretica, 49*(1), 53-59.

Campbell, M. L., & Guzman, J. A. (2003). Impact of a proactive approach to improve end-of-life care in a medical ICU. *CHEST Journal, 123*(1), 266-271.

Clark, Carolyn (1993). Adult Education Research Annual Conference (AERC) Proceedings (34th, University Park, Pennsylvania, May 1993).

Cohen, R. (2013, August). Sugar Love: A Not So Sweet Tale. *National Geographic, 224*(2), 78-97.

Conner, K., & Malmin, K. (1983). *The Covenants- The Key to God's Relationship with Mankind,* City Bible Publishing, Portland, Oregon.

Cornelissen, G., & Otsuka, K. (2016). Chronobiology of Aging: A Mini-Review. *Gerontology.*

Cowen, G.P. (2003). Heart. *Holman, Illustrated Bible Dictionary.* Holman Bible Publishers, Nashville, Tenn.

Crowe, F. L., Appleby, P. N., Travis, R. C., & Key, T. J. (2013). Risk of hospitalization or death from ischemic heart disease among British vegetarians and nonvegetarians: results from the EPIC-Oxford cohort study.*The American journal of clinical nutrition, 97*(3), 597-603

Davies, P. (1983). *God and the new physics.* Simon and Schuster.

Dean, R. J. (2003). Joy. *Holman, Illustrated Bible Dictionary.* Holman Bible Publishers, Nashville, Tenn.

Dersh, J., Gatchel, R. J., Mayer, T., Polatin, P., & Temple, O. R. (2006). Prevalence of psychiatric disorders in patients with chronic disabling occupational spinal disorders. Spine, 31(10),1156-1162.

Drummond, Henry. (1883/2008). *Natural Law in the Spiritual World*. Radford, Va: Wilder Publications.

Earley, D. (2008). *Prayer: The Timeless Secret of High-Impact Leaders*. Living Ink Books, Chattanooga, Tenn.

Erickson, M. J. (1998). *Christian Theology*. Grand Rapids, MI: Baker Book House.

Esmer, G., Blum, J., Rulf, J., & Pier, J. (2010). Mindfulness-based stress reduction for failed back surgery syndrome: a randomized controlled trial. *The Journal of the American Osteopathic Association, 110*(11), 646-652.

Estruch, R., Ros, E., Salas-Salvadó, J., Covas, M. I., Corella, D., Arós, F., ... & Lamuela-Raventos, R. M. (2013). Primary prevention of cardiovascular disease with a Mediterranean diet. *New England Journal of Medicine,368*(14), 1279-1290.

Féart, C., Samieri, C., Rondeau, V., Amieva, H., Portet, F., Dartigues, J. F., ... & Barberger-Gateau, P. (2009). Adherence to a Mediterranean diet, cognitive decline, and risk of dementia. *Jama, 302*(6), 638-648.

Feinberg, J. S. (2005). Theodicy. *Elwell's Evangelical Dictionary of Theology (2nd ed.)*. Grand Rapids, Mich.: Baker Book House.

Flint-Wagner, H. G., Lisse, J., Lohman, T. G., Going, S. B., Guido, T., Cussler, E., ... & Yocum, D. E. (2009). Assessment of a sixteen-week training program on strength, pain, and function in rheumatoid arthritis patients. *JCR: Journal of Clinical Rheumatology, 15*(4), 165-171

Foster, R. J. (1988). *Celebration of discipline: the path to spiritual growth*. San Francisco: Harper & Row.

Gassen, N. C., Chrousos, G. P., Binder, E. B., & Zannas, A. S. (2016). Life stress, glucocorticoid signaling, and the aging epigenome: Implications for aging-related diseases. *Neuroscience & Biobehavioral Reviews*.

Gibbons, Patrick (2009, March), Chronic Pain and Psychiatric Symptoms. *Update Addiction Medicine*, Congdon Lecture Series, Grand Blanc, Mi.

Galbraith, M. W. (1990). *Adult learning methods: A guide for effective instruction*. Krieger Publishing Company, Krieger Drive, Malabar, FL 32950.

Garcia, A. M. (2013). State laws regulating prescribing of controlled substances: balancing the public health problems of chronic pain and prescription painkiller abuse and overdose. *The Journal of Law, Medicine & Ethics, 41*(s1), 42-45.

Geisler, N. (2004). *Systematic Theology, Vol. Three*, Bloomington, Minn: Bethany House Publishers.

Grider, K.L. (2005). Heaven. *Elwell's Evangelical Dictionary ofTheology (2nd ed.)*. Grand Rapids, Mich.: Baker Book House.

Grossman, M. (2006). *Unprotected: a campus psychiatrist reveals how political correctness in her profession endangers every student*. New York, New York; Penguin Group.

Guthrie, Donald. (2005), John. *New Bible Commentary*. InterVarsity Press, Downers Grove, Il.

Hakim, A. A., Petrovitch, H., Burchfiel, C. M., Ross, G. W.,

Rodriguez, B. L., White, L. R., ... & Abbott, R. D. (1998). Effects of walking on mortality among nonsmoking retired men. *New England Journal of Medicine, 338*(2), 94-99.

Henry, M. (1961). *Matthew Henry's commentary in one volume.* Zondervan Publishing House.

Hoekema, A. (1994). *Created in God's image.* Grand Rapids, Mich.: Eerdmans.

Holton, E. F., Swanson, R. A., & Naquin, S. S. (2001). Andragogy in practice: Clarifying the Andragogical model of adult learning. *Performance Improvement Quarterly, 14*(1), 118-143.

Höfle, M., Hauck, M., Engel, A. K., & Senkowski, D. (2012). Viewing a needle pricking a hand that you perceive as yours enhances unpleasantness of pain. *PAIN®, 153*(5), 1074-1081.

Holy Bible: Today's New International Version. (2005). Colorado Springs, CO: International Bible Society.

Horwitz, A. V., & Wakefield, J. C. (2007). *The loss of sadness: How psychiatry transformed normal sorrow into depressive disorder.* Oxford University Press.

Kasapis, C., & Thompson, P. D. (2005). The effects of physical activity on serum C-reactive protein and inflammatory markers: a systematic review. *Journal of the American College of Cardiology, 45*(10), 1563-1569.

Keener, C. S. (1993). *The IVP Bible Background Commentary: New Testament.* InterVarsity Press.

Keller, H. (1980). *The Story of My Life.* Watermill Press, Mahwah, New Jersey.

Kinzbrunner, B. M. (2004). Jewish medical ethics and end-of-life care. *Journal of Palliative Medicine*, *7*(4), 558-573.

Kokkinos, P., Myers, J., Kokkinos, J. P., Pittaras, A., Narayan, P., Manolis, A., ... & Singh, S. (2008). Exercise capacity and mortality in black and white men. *Circulation*, *117*(5), 614-622.

Kurtz, S., Ong, K., Lau, E., Mowat, F., & Halpern, M. (2007). Projections of primary and revision hip and knee arthroplasty in the United States from 2005 to 2030. *J Bone Joint Surg Am*, *89*(4), 780-785.

Kurth, Don (2006, May), Office Evaluation of the Addicted Patient. *Update Addiction Medicine*, Congdon Lecture Series, Grand Blanc, Mi

Ladd, G.E. (2005). Kingdom of Christ, God, Heaven. *Terminology. Elwell's Evangelical Dictionary of Theology (2nd ed.).* Grand Rapids, Mich.: Baker Book House

Lichtman, J. H., Froelicher, E. S., Blumenthal, J. A., Carney, R. M., Doering, L. V., Frasure-Smith, N., ... & Vaccarino, V. (2014). Depression as a risk factor for poor prognosis among patients with acute coronary syndrome: systematic review and recommendations a scientific statement from the American Heart Association. *Circulation*, *129*(12), 1350-1369.

Lewis, C. S. (1940), *The Problem of Pain,* HarperCollins Publishers, Inc., New York, New York.

Lewis, C. S. (1942). The Screwtape Letters. *Geoffrey Bles, United Kingdom.*

Lewis, C. S. (1952/2001). Mere Christianity. *San Francisco: Harper, SanFrancisco.*

Lin, A. L., Coman, D., Jiang, L., Rothman, D. L., & Hyder, F. (2014). Caloric restriction impedes age-related decline of mitochondrial function and neuronal activity. *Journal of Cerebral Blood Flow & Metabolism, 34*(9), 1440-1443.

Lumeng, J. C., Miller, A., Peterson, K. E., Kaciroti, N., Sturza, J., Rosenblum, K., & Vazquez, D. M. (2014). Diurnal cortisol pattern, eating behaviors and overweight in low-income preschool-aged children. *Appetite,73,* 65-72.

Macchia, S. A. (1999). Becoming a Healthy Church. *Grand Rapids: Baker.*

Magee, B. (2001). *The Story of Philosophy.* New York, NY: DK Publishing Inc.

Margolis, R. (2013). Educational Differences in Healthy Behavior Changes and Adherence Among Middle-aged Americans. *Journal of Health and Social Behavior, 54*(3), 353–368.

Manson, J. E., Greenland, P., LaCroix, A. Z., Stefanick, M. L., Mouton, C. P., Oberman, A., ... & Siscovick, D. S. (2002). Walking compared with vigorous exercise for the prevention of cardiovascular events in women. *New England Journal of Medicine, 347*(10), 716-725.

McCarroll, Brian D.O. (2011, March). Lecture on *Benzodiazepine Abuse-Prescribing Pitfalls and Pearls for the Primary Care Physician,* Congdon Lecture Series, Grand Blanc, MI.

McCarthy, L. H., Bigal, M. E., Katz, M., Derby, C., & Lipton, R. B. (2009). Chronic pain and obesity in elderly people: results from the Einstein aging study. *Journal of the American Geriatrics Society, 57*(1), 115-119.

McLaren, N. (2010). Toward an osteopathic psychiatry: the

biocognitive model of mind. *The Journal of the American Osteopathic Association, 110*(12), 725-732.

Merriam, S. B., Caffarella, R. S., & Baumgartner, L. M. (2007). *Learning in adulthood: A comprehensive guide.* John Wiley & Sons.

Messier, S. P., Mihalko, S. L., Legault, C., Miller, G. D., Nicklas, B. J., DeVita, P., ... & Williamson, J. D. (2013). Effects of intensive diet and exercise on knee joint loads, inflammation, and clinical outcomes among overweight and obese adults with knee osteoarthritis: the IDEA randomized clinical trial. *Jama, 310*(12), 1263-1273.

Mezirow, J. (1997). Transformative learning: Theory to practice. *New directions for adult and continuing education, 1997*(74), 5-12.

Miller, A. H., Maletic, V., & Raison, C. L. (2009). Inflammation and its discontents: the role of cytokines in the pathophysiology of major depression. *Biological psychiatry, 65*(9), 732-741.

Motyer, J.A. (2005), Psalms 119. *New Bible Commentary.* InterVarsity Press, Downers Grove, Il.

Munroe, M. (2004). *Rediscovering the kingdom: ancient hope for our 21st century world.* Shippensburg, PA: Destiny Image

Nedley, N. (2001). *Depression: The way out.* Ardmore, OK: Nedley Pub.

O'Leary, A. (1985). Self-efficacy and health. *Behaviour research and therapy,23*(4), 437-45

Orlich, M. J., Singh, P. N., Sabaté, J., Jaceldo-Siegl, K., Fan, J., Knutsen, S., ... & Fraser, G. E. (2013). Vegetarian dietary patterns and mortality in Adventist Health Study 2. *JAMA internal medicine, 173*(13), 1230-1238.

Ornish, D., Brown, S. E., Billings, J. H., Scherwitz, L. W., Armstrong, W. T., Ports, T. A., ... & Brand, R. J. (1990). Can lifestyle changes reverse coronary heart disease?: The Lifestyle Heart Trial. *The Lancet, 336*(8708), 129-133.

Ornish, D., Magbanua, M. J. M., Weidner, G., Weinberg, V., Kemp, C., Green, C., ... & Haqq, C. M. (2008). Changes in prostate gene expression in men undergoing an intensive nutrition and lifestyle intervention. *Proceedings of the National Academy of Sciences, 105*(24), 8369-8374.

Orozco-Solis, R., & Sassone-Corsi, P. (2014). Circadian clock: linking epigenetics to aging. *Current opinion in genetics & development, 26*, 66-72.

Osterhaven, M. E. (2005). Spirit. *Elwell's Evangelical Dictionary of Theology (2nd ed.)*. Grand Rapids, Mich.: Baker Book House.

Otto, A. (2011, September 27). Rigorous Exercise May Delay Hip Replacement. *Rheumatology News*.

Overman, C. L., Bossema, E. R., van Middendorp, H., Wijngaards-de Meij, L., Verstappen, S. M., Bulder, M., ... & Geenen, R. (2012). The prospective association between psychological distress and disease activity in rheumatoid arthritis: a multilevel regression analysis. *Annals of the rheumatic diseases, 71*(2), 192-197.

Packer, J. L. (2005). Regeneration. *Elwell's Evangelical Dictionary of Theology (2nd ed.)*. Grand Rapids, Mich.: Baker Book House.

Pascual-Leone, A., Rubio, B., Pallardó, F., & Catalá, M. D. (1996).

Rapid-rate transcranial magnetic stimulation of left dorsolateral prefrontal cortex in drug-resistant depression. *The Lancet, 348*(9022), 233-237.

Pan, A., Sun, Q., Okereke, O. I., Rexrode, K. M., & Hu, F. B. (2011). Depression and risk of stroke morbidity and mortality: a meta-analysis and systematic review. *Jama, 306*(11), 1241-1249.

Puchalski, C., Ferrell, B., Virani, R., Otis-Green, S., Baird, P., Bull, J., ... & Pugliese, K. (2009). Improving the quality of spiritual care as a dimension of palliative care: the report of the Consensus Conference. *Journal of palliative medicine, 12*(10), 885-904.

Pratt, D. D. (1998). *Five Perspectives on Teaching in Adult and Higher Education.* Krieger Publishing Co., PO Box 9542, Melbourne, FL 32902-9542.

Qi, Q., Chu, A. Y., Kang, J. H., Jensen, M. K., Curhan, G. C., Pasquale, L. R., ... & Chasman, D. I. (2012). Sugar-sweetened beverages and genetic risk of obesity. *New England Journal of Medicine, 367*(15), 1387-1396.

Ratey, J. J. (2001). *A user's guide to the brain: Perception, attention, and the four theatres of the brain.* Vintage.

Rubak, S., Sandbæk, A., Lauritzen, T., & Christensen, B. (2005). Motivational interviewing: a systematic review and meta-analysis. *Br J Gen Pract, 55*(513), 305-312.

Rasmussen, H. N., Scheier, M. F., & Greenhouse, J. B. (2009). Optimism and physical health: A meta-analytic review. *Annals of behavioral medicine,37*(3), 239-256.

Robinson, H. W. (1947). *The Christian Doctrine of Man,* (3rd ed.). Edinburgh, SCT: T. & T. Clark.

Sandin, R.T. (1987), One of the Best Teachers of the Church, *Christian History*, 6(15), 26-29.

Scott, J. J. (2004). *Jewish backgrounds of the New Testament.* Grand Rapids, MI: Baker Books.

Sears, B. (1999). *The anti-aging zone.* New York, NY: Regan Books, an imprint of HarperCollins.

Seminowicz, D. A., Wideman, T. H., Naso, L., Hatami-Khoroushahi, Z., Fallatah, S., Ware, M. A., ... & Stone, L. S. (2011). Effective treatment of chronic low back pain in humans reverses abnormal brain anatomy and function. *The Journal of neuroscience, 31*(20), 7540-7550.

Shimbo, D., Chaplin, W., Crossman, D., Haas, D., & Davidson, K. W. (2005). Role of depression and inflammation in incident coronary heart disease events. *The American journal of cardiology, 96*(7), 1016-1021.

Shreeve, James, "What's in Your Mind," *National Geographic Magazine,* March 2005, p2.

Spiceland, J. D. (2005). Theodicy. *Elwell's Evangelical Dictionary of Theology (2nd ed.).* Grand Rapids, Mich.: Baker Book House.

Stanaway, F. F., Gnjidic, D., Blyth, F. M., Le Couteur, D. G., Naganathan, V., Waite, L., ... & Cumming, R. G. (2011). How fast does the Grim Reaper walk? Receiver operating characteristics curve analysis in healthy men aged 70 and over. *Bmj, 343,* d7679.

Studenski, S., Perera, S., Patel, K., Rosano, C., Faulkner, K., Inzitari, M., ... & Nevitt, M. (2011). Gait speed and survival in older adults. *Jama, 305*(1), 50-58.

Suji, G., & Sivakami, S. (2004). Glucose, glycation and aging. *Biogerontology*, *5*(6), 365-373.

Svege, I., Nordsletten, L., Fernandes, L., & Risberg, M. A. (2013). Exercise therapy may postpone total hip replacement surgery in patients with hip osteoarthritis: a long-term follow-up of a randomised trial. *Annals of the rheumatic diseases*, annrheumdis-2013.

Tompson, T., Benz, J., Agiesta, J., Brewer, K. H., Bye, L., Reimer, R., & Junius, D. (2012). Obesity in the United States: public perceptions. *The food industry*, *53*(26), 21.

Towns, E. L., Stetzer, E., & Bird, W. (2007). 11 innovations in the local church: how today's leaders can learn, discern and move into the future. Ventura, CA: Regal Books.

Tozer, A.W., (1948/2010) *The Pursuit of God*, Alba & Tromm: Las Vegas, Neveda.

Transformative learning. (2017, February 2). In *Wikipedia, The Free Encyclopedia*. Retrieved 18:50, June 3, 2017

Turk, D. C., Wilson, H. D., & Cahana, A. (2011). Treatment of chronic non-cancer pain. *The Lancet*, *377*(9784), 2226-2235.

Vella, J. (2002). *Learning to listen, learning to teach: The power of dialogue in educating adults*. John Wiley & Sons.

Vemuri, P., Lesnick, T. G., Przybelski, S. A., Machulda, M., Knopman, D. S., Mielke, M. M., ... & Jack, C. R. (2014). Association of lifetime intellectual enrichment with cognitive decline in the older population. *JAMA neurology*, *71*(8), 1017-1024.

Von Drehle, David (2014, August 18). Manopause?! Aging, Insecurity and the $2 Billion Testosterone Industry. Time, 184(6), 38.

Wade, G. J. (2011). Rethinking the model of osteoarthritis: a clinical viewpoint. *The Journal of the American Osteopathic Association, 111*(11), 631-637.

Walsh, D. A., & Radcliffe, J. C. (2002). Pain beliefs and perceived physical disability of patients with chronic low back pain. *Pain, 97*(1), 23-31.

White, E. G. (2004). *To Be Like Jesus*. Review and Herald Pub Assoc.

Wiseman, M. (2008). The second World Cancer Research Fund/American Institute for Cancer Research expert report. Food, nutrition, physical activity, and the prevention of cancer: a global perspective. *Proceedings of the Nutrition Society, 67*(03), 253-256.

Willette, A. A., Bendlin, B. B., Starks, E. J., Birdsill, A. C., Johnson, S. C., Christian, B. T., ... & Jonaitis, E. M. (2015). Association of insulin resistance with cerebral glucose uptake in late middle–aged adults at risk for Alzheimer disease. *JAMA neurology, 72*(9), 1013-1020.

Williams, D. A., & Thorn, B. E. (1989). An empirical assessment of pain beliefs. *Pain, 36*(3), 351-358.

Whitmer, R. A., Gustafson, D. R., Barrett-Connor, E., Haan, M.N., Gunderson, E. P., & Yaffe, K. (2008). Central obesity and increased risk of dementia more than three decades later. *Neurology, 71*(14), 1057-1064.

Yaffe, K., Lindquist, K., Schwartz, A. V., Vitartas, C., Vittinghoff, E., Satterfield, S., ... & Harris, T. (2011). Advanced glycation end product level, diabetes, and accelerated cognitive aging. *Neurology, 77*(14), 1351-1356.

Yokell, M. A., Delgado, M. K., Zaller, N. D., Wang, N. E., McGowan, S. K., & Green, T. C. (2014). Presentation of prescription and nonprescription opioid overdoses to US emergency departments. *JAMA internal medicine,174*(12), 2034-2037

Young, S. (2004). *Jesus calling: Enjoying peace in His presence: Devotions for every day of the year*. Nashville: Integrity.

Zannas, A. S., & West, A. E. (2014). Epigenetics and the regulation of stress vulnerability and resilience. *Neuroscience, 264*, 157-170

Made in the USA
Columbia, SC
28 January 2018